Connect to Sleep

Theory and Neuroscience of Gentle Bedtimes

0-12 months

HELEN STEVENS

First published by Busybird Publishing 2019

Copyright © 2019 Helen Stevens

ISBN 978-1-925585-68-1

This book is copyright. Apart from any fair dealing for the purposes of study, research, criticism, review, or as otherwise permitted under the Copyright Act, no part may be reproduced by any process without written permission. Enquiries should be made through the publisher.

Baby photographer; Beckie Littler. Stylist. www.beckielittler.com
Baby images courtesy of Rupert

Typesetting: Busybird Publishing

www.busybird.com.au

This book is testament to the power of unyielding support and love of family, friends and colleagues, my heart-filled thanks.

If it were not for the families themselves, their stories and messages, I would never be able to appreciate how far I have to go, and how far I have come.

To every struggling parent I can only say, thank you and have hope, because one day, you too, will see your babies bloom, and all those moments of doubt will melt away as your children grow to young adults who become more than you could have ever hoped for.

Love you Sammie and Matt.

Contents

A word from the author	i
Preface	v
Introduction	ix
Thinking about Parents	1
Thinking about Babies	7
Communication	13
Noah's family story	17
Avi's family story	31
Ayaz's family story	47
Charlotte's family story	61
Be kind to yourself; allow your intuition to grow	77
Daily sleep hours GUIDE	79
References	83
About the Author	91

Reviews

"Babies are individuals from the very beginning, but it can be hard for parents to easily read and understand their newborn baby. Helen Stevens has written a wonderful book taking us through the journey of the newborn baby and his and her parents as they negotiate a way of understanding each other, particularly in relation to sleep. Helen's approach shows great respect for the baby as a person and for parents as people with their own rich inner world worlds. Helen demonstrates the power of an individualised approach to helping babies develop a relationship based system of self-regulation: sleeping, waking, feeding, playing by being with people who are available and responding in a contingent way to the baby subtle cues. Building on an understanding of the neurobiology of early infant development, using a vivid, but very typical, set of family stories around babies and sleep Helen helps us into the world of the baby and of the parents.

I believe this humane approach in this book to helping babies develop comfortable corregulation with their parents and others has a huge amount to offer all parents. This book has the capacity to help parents feel that they are able to love their babies and provide the necessary response of structure to help them become creative and organised persons! Parents and professionals alike will find in this book a gentle but firm pathway through the earliest period of the young child's life."

> Associate Professor Campbell Paul, Consultant Infant Psychiatrist, Royal Children's Hospital and the Royal Women's Hospital Melbourne. Coordinator, Master of Mental Health Sciences, Infant Stream, Department of Psychiatry University of Melbourne.

"New parents can find themselves in the fog of sleep-deprivation, desperate for effective sleep-strategies, only to then be advised to use 'tough-love' sleep-strategies on their beautiful new baby. Having worked alongside Australia's infant sleep 'Guru', Helen Stevens, over many years, I have seen the relief on the faces of parents and professionals when she guides them in how parents can safely and gently settle their babies to sleep.

Helen's new book offers a wealth of information about babies and parenting but is easy to read because it takes the reader through stories with real parents and babies and how their problems were remedied with kind and loving sleep-settling strategies that improved the parent-infant relationship, rather than promoting extended separation and crying. You can feel the relief and joy in the parents' stories of how Helen guided them through tough times into a positive and loving experience as mums and dads. This is the sleep-solutions book that I recommend to new parents."

Timothy O'Leary, Therapist, Educator and Author; *Dads Who Can.*

"As a parent of two it is impossible to say how important Helen's work is. As a psychologist, I knew all the theory, but societal pressure to do some form of controlled crying was enormous. As a terribly sleep deprived family we had given up hope of ever sleeping while we had young children. The arrival of our second baby really pushed us to the limit of exhaustion. With our toddler, we had previously done controlled comforting, when she was 10 months, it was awful, but we followed the plan exactly as the family Centre had coached us, in desperation. Again at 2 years, with support from our paediatrician we tried it again. It was horrible but we were desperate so caved in to pressure from our paediatrician, local doctor, family and friends. After that we committed to not doing that ever again, nor have we. My child and family health nurse recommended I speak with Helen. OUR WORLD CHANGED from that very first call. It all made so much sense, she clearly knew the theory, and her knowledge and kindness were so comforting. Not once were our heart strings stretched like they had been when we did the 'tough love' approach. We offered BOTH our children experiences that were loving and gentle and they both slept better, much better. Just over one year after contact with Helen we all still sleep, and often talk about the time our lives were changed! Our only regret is that we let societal pressure get us with our first child. By being encouraged to connect with our children and offer them love and kindness, we were able to move away from the 'get your baby to sleep for your sake' mentality, to a much more comfortable way of supporting our children to sleep."

Dr Ruth Gardener. Clinical Psychologist, wife and mother of 2.

A word from the author

As individuals, we are all vastly different. We respond differently and we think differently to all other individuals. However, difficulties can arise despite the best of intentions. With my first baby, I cuddled, loved and cuddled her some more. My heart swelled with the love I felt. Within that cloud, I loved and cuddled her to sleep. I adored the sense of us being as one, but it became increasingly obvious that she had her own needs, her individual needs and I was at risk of blanketing her in love, so much so that she began to struggle to sleep.

My hugs were less needed as she became more able to move around and adjust herself. What started to become clear was that I was doing everything for her. It felt rewarding to me, but she needed a relationship that supported her in gaining a little space and it was difficult for me to see this until she really protested. I had become such an intensely loving parent, I had forgotten to look to her for cues of readiness to reach out to her world, because I was so engrossed in bringing it all to her to make it easier for her. It was within this space that I was no longer addressing her needs, but my own.

She showed me through her sleep struggles, that she needed a relationship with a parent who watched for her cues, and waited to see what she needed, rather than to impose what I thought she needed. The difference was her continued growth in a warm loving relationship, allowing her to express herself, and me providing for her needs. It was within this new relationship that sleep began to find its way.

Baby two was as intensely loved but right from the start his cues and communications were respected. The care I offered him was based on his emotions and needs; resulting in a happy baby and an intensely rewarding experience, even at sleep time.

Twenty years on, and thousands upon thousands of families later, we know it is the infant-parent relationship that scaffolds the baby's growth, through contingent care and connection; that's what really counts. So, the interaction that flows between each individual infant and parent is based on the cues and clues that babies offer that indicate their emotions and social needs.

Simply put, a baby needs a relationship with their parent or caregiver, who sees the baby for who they are, and provides care in response to those individual baby's cues [1]. The job of the parent is to fine tune looking, thinking and feeling about their baby and the baby's experiences, so they can provide synchronised care. The job of the baby is to cue needs and to develop a relationship, or attachment, to someone who can provide this care. This in-tune relationship, or quality relationship, is what we are striving for - care that matches the cues [2,3]. If we look for and respect what is happening within the baby, the baby's brain, and our relationships with our babies, we can unlock many of the mysteries that underpin the early years' challenges.

Within this book are family stories viewed through the lens of current knowledge and understanding. This approach offers some simple, kind yet effective ways to help babies find sleep while being offered parental care and guidance. With respect to each family, the individuals within each family, and the unique infant-parent relationships that have developed, these stories offer a window into the world of baby behaviours and highlight some things to consider when similar situations arise within other families.

At no time do these stories assume to present the complete world of the family in context. Every person comes to parenting with a life, a story, different to another. This is the context into which a baby is born. The parent, the parent's pre-baby life, expectations and experiences will, in some way, influence how this infant-parent relationship flows. For the baby, from anticipation, to conception, inter-uterine exposures, DNA, temperament, and life experiences, each daily experience will influence the ebb and flow of the development of the infant 'self' and how each individual baby responds to the world around them [4]. These are all very important considerations when thinking about a baby who, for whatever reason, is unable to calm for or stay asleep. When a baby cannot sleep, it may be as simple as the result of a bubble of wind, or it may be something more, much more. It is hoped parents are able to consider the world in which their babies are growing, to be reflective about the baby, the baby's experiences within the context of their individual family, and to think more widely than about just getting a baby to sleep.

The follow stories are commonly seen in my practice and may therefore resonate with parents in a way that may trigger some uncomfortable feelings. If that happens, it may be timely to consider speaking with someone who can offer you support, so you can enjoy this very precious and short lived phase of life. This is the time of life to recognise and address triggers so you can get on with being the kind of parent you want to be and are not still trying to sort your own life while you are parenting an adolescent!

Preface

"Transitioning infants to sleep, respectfully"

Some express concern that comforting babies in their transition to sleep will lead to babies who are unable to develop the skill of falling to sleep without their parents. It is often asked, *How can picking up an unsettled or crying baby help them learn to settle to sleep more easily?* Or, *How is it that staying with a baby while they fall to sleep will help them develop better sleep habits?*

There are those who advocate that letting babies 'work it out alone' at sleep time is a means by which they learn to be more capable and independent. In the light of what is known of infant developmental needs, leaving a distressed baby alone at any time, be it sleep time or not, is not supportive of emerging self-dependence.

Supporting a baby involves cuddling and comforting, so if you want your baby to sleep well, they firstly need to learn how to calm and be calmed by another. Teaching a baby to sleep well without a parent seems opposing to what is needed to learn about calming for sleep. Driving this message to leave your baby to self-settle, even if he cries for quite a bit, is the idea that this short period of distress, alone and uncomforted, is a small price to pay for the outcome of good sleep habits. The premise is that if a baby is left to cry at sleep time, they will be able to sleep for longer and longer periods and as well as settle to sleep readily. The message is then, even though it is difficult for parents, even counterintuitive, to listen and not support your crying baby, it is suggested that crying alone at sleep time is a necessary step toward better sleep patterns. This approach looks beyond the actual distress periods at sleep times, presuming that once you and your baby are sleeping, then everything will fall back into a better place. The assumption being, the end result is more important than the experience for the parent-baby connection. In the description of controlled comforting and controlled crying itself, of leaving a distressed baby alone to cry, even for short periods, seems contrary to the social and emotional needs of the developing baby.

The stories you are about to read are from families who shared their experiences when they reached out for help with their infants' sleep. All of these families had tried many means of promoting sleep and calm, some of which involved leaving infants to settle themselves. These stories speak of infants struggling both when transitioning to sleep and maintaining sleep. Illustrated in the change to more peaceful sleep transitions is the power of contingent, responsive care.

Helen Stevens invites the reader to step back from the message that infants should learn to settle themselves to sleep, and consider a broader picture and a different approach. The shared stories are ways of thinking about the infant-parent experience, make clear the importance of recognising, even when we are very tired, that babies do all they can to tell us what they need.

As I read each story – each beginning with chaotic and challenging sleep patterns and strained interactions, and ending with easy transitions to sleep and more peaceful babies and parents – I could not help but think, *If only parents didn't think picking up their baby was harmful, how much more free they would be to read and respond to babies' cues.*

What Helen illustrates in this approach, and in the reasoning for each thought, is that a mismatch between infant needs and what parents think helpful, often leads to challenging and exhausting outcomes. Each family's story illustrates parents' uncertainty that something so simple as considering infant communication – watching for their infants' cues and fostering that powerful connection – could help change their struggles around sleep. Yet in each follow-up with families, parents report how this way of thinking *did* make a difference, and themes of understanding their baby and deepening the infant-parent relationship were apparent.

What we, as readers, can take away is that an understanding of the critical role of caregiving that promotes the connection for both infant and parent, in conjunction with simple changes, illustrates the success of settling infants to sleep with contingent, responsive care. What we see, also, is the renewed connection and joy shared between the parents and their babies. With this, Helen helps us to see that learning more about infants' social and emotional needs and communication, can result in longer hours of sleep *without crying*."

   – Associate Professor Wendy Middlemiss
   Department of Educational Psychology
   University of North Texas.

Introduction

When babies struggle to sleep, the flow on effects are real for the entire family. With this book I hope to provide families with an understanding of what influences the settling for the sleep process and sleep maintenance. Hopefully this information will, in turn, help families move forward when sleep struggles are tipping the joy and love of babies into exhaustion and often, understandable, helplessness and frustration. Research has provided us with a world of information about babies' brains as well as the importance of infant-parent relationships in the development of optimal emotional, social and even physical development as a foundation for life [5,6,7,8].

These stories are real. They come from contact with families who are really struggling with baby sleep challenges. These stories have been generously shared by families who are happy to have their experience shared, in the hope that in some way it can be helpful to others who are feeling overwhelmed. Although deidentified for privacy reasons, these stories are often not very different for the repeated themes I have witnessed over 20 years of specialising in this area.

As a professional resource, this book supports families in a kind and respectful way, to guide, soothe and comfort babies at sleep time. Baby sleep has been a contentious topic for as many years as I have been involved with families struggling with sleep. Families often report that a commonly supported method of 'getting' babies to sleep for longer periods is distressing for their baby and themselves because it promotes increasing parental absence to help the baby sleep. With the knowledge of family relationships and how the infant brain, mind and body function, clinicians are also keen to offer parents sleep promotion education and information that encourage parents to think about the infant's experience and to respond to each individual infant's communication. This process encourages parents to be more present and to be contingently responding to their child's cues and communication [8,9].

Babies can be supported in a sensitive way that achieves longer sleep periods without needing the once often recommended sleep training of 'controlled crying' and modifications of controlled crying including controlled comforting [10]. Controlled crying methods promote increasing parental absence, infant stress, and unmet baby needs for comfort and care during the transition to sleep [11].

From a relational and infant mental health and wellbeing perspective, I do not advocate for parental absence from distressed babies, nor do I promote sleep for periods that are not normal for a baby. Instead, I encourage parents to understand how their babies' brains function, and how best to provide kind and contingent care in response to the cues and behaviours of each individual baby. That way, even at sleep time, the quality of the interaction between the baby and caregivers is maintained.

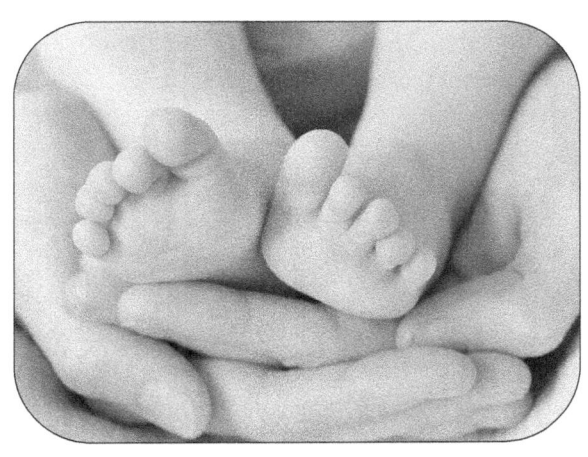

Chapter 1
Thinking about Parents

Nothing can prepare for the reality of parenting. One thing that is clear to me is that the 'perfect parent' only ever exists in the mind of those who are thinking about and anticipating parenting. 'Real parenting' is born with the baby. It very quickly becomes reality that parents can only do their best, which means parenting when tired, unsure, confused and often overwhelmed. The ideal world of parenting gives way to reality when a baby is born. Not only can this be quite a shock to new parents, it is compounded by everyone, mostly well-wishers, telling them how to do it better. As kind as these intentions can be from friends and family, it can result in the erosion of the parents' emerging confidence in their ability to make decisions for the welfare of their baby and their family.

Being the 'good enough' or 'ordinary mother' as paediatrician and psychoanalysis in the 1950's, Dr Winnicott termed it, is a much more realistic aim [12], or what I call 'a normal parent'. Parenting is learning on the job. It's not a completed art form; rather, it is ongoing evolution and growth. Parenting is trial and error, with the main emphasis being on trying again. Learning on the job means not getting it right all the time, but from that comes the opportunity to learn. Parenting allows for numerous 'learning' experiences. Keep trying and skills will develop.

Babies are the least judgmental beings we could possibly hope for. All they want is to connect with someone who will provide them with a sense of safety and protection, and of course to provide for all the physical requirements as well. Without their emotional and social needs being met, a baby struggles to grow to thrive, or even learn trust. A baby needs many things to become a regulated, emotionally and socially competent adult. They need someone who they can form a relationship with that provides protection, comfort and a sense of self-worth and belonging. [13,14]. Nothing will ever flow perfectly in life because we are humans and that is not an exacting form. There will be many stressors in life, yet when your baby experiences times when there is a disruption within their relationship with you, and if that is then followed by efforts to repair the disruption, that helps babies prepare for life. The baby then learns how inevitable relationship ruptures can be repaired, which is all part of building their adaptation to stress [15]. As parents, we do make mistakes and will often get it wrong, but the important thing is to keep trying.

Our life is not a series of smooth flowing events and experiences, rather, life is filled with ups and downs, and so is a baby's life. Therefore, it is critical to bookend those experiences with love and compassionate, contingent care. Parents are often their own greatest critics, and mostly undeservedly. Rather than rejoicing the achievements, parents can become stuck in self-criticism and self-doubt which breeds feelings of hopelessness, that can become a self-fulfilling prophecy. In this state, parents often can't see what is being done well, but instead focus on self-judgement when those inevitable mismatches of communication occur.

Parents can become stuck thinking about their own competence, rather than accepting that we all adjust to parenthood and become increasingly skilled over time. If you can be kind to yourself and considerate of your baby, you are doing well. Cherish even the tiniest of achievements. Given the opportunity, babies develop a strong and lasting bond with their parents. So, when you are self-doubting, keep in mind, all your baby wants is you; you with all your perceived imperfections. Your baby sees you as perfectly you and they want for nothing more.

Being a parent is a tough gig, but no parent is alone in those feelings, despite the times when a sense of isolation can creep in. Most parents feel uncertain to some extent as they strive to be the best parent they can be, so if self-doubt or anxiety are interfering with you achieving that goal, then it is important to reach for the supports around you so you can normalise the ups and downs of parenting. These variations don't go away. We just learn to manage them better. If you are struggling, be sure you chat with your family, friends, nurse or doctor. Have a look around for a supportive parent group, because parents supporting parents has the potential to become a life line for new parents.

There is a well understood phenomenon that occurs when the going gets tough in parenting; relationships take a hit. It can be the adult relationship or the infant-parent relationship or relationships with extended family and friends. This is more common than people realise. It happens because humans are social beings and are inclined to lean on the ones we love most when we are struggling. Parenting adds new and often frustrating dimensions to relationships, and together with the inevitable sleep deprivation, cracks can begin to show. What parents often find helpful is to be as open as possible when rifts occur. Acknowledge, discuss and look for pathways forward, rather than becoming defensive, resentful and critical. This only causes a greater divide between you and the ones you need around you. If parents can parent in partnership with each other, or a single parent in partnership with a close friend or family, it provides the scaffolding for the growth to strengthen that relationship rather than continuing the strain.

Parenting is not easy. The new challenges often feel overwhelming. We need supports in some form or another to help get through the inevitable times when things just don't go to plan. Allow your relationships to grow stronger as the result of this enormous adjustment phase; grow with it. Working together does not always mean agreeing, it means respecting the other's experiences, listening and trying to find the ground where you can make this all work long term. The adjustment phase is the most challenging because you will have to adapt to the sleeplessness, the lack of flexibility and the additional two hours it takes just to go for a coffee!

Remember you weren't attracted to your partner because they mirrored you. Most likely you have very different traits and personalities and, in fact, you're partnered because your individual characteristics complement each other. That all sounds very romantic until you begin to parent. It is then that you become acutely aware of how differently you see things. We learn how to parent as a result of our experiences. If you were parented with a gentle, cuddling parent and your partner had a parent who was distant, and thought that affection would result in a 'soft child', then these differences will probably become amplified in the presence of a newborn baby. Try to infuse a sense of humor and respect for each other's opinion into your partnership, to help soften the inevitable prickly times [16].

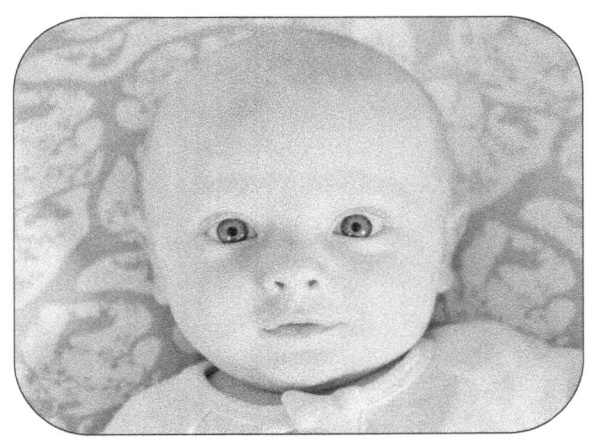

Chapter 2
Thinking about Babies

In the moment of doing all the 'things' necessary for a baby, it can be easy to forget that the baby is so much more than someone who demands of you physically. Babies are entities unto themselves, they are a 'self' and their experiences impact on how the 'self' develops [17,18].

When you were born, you were not a different person to who you are now. You are just a baby who has grown with many, many experiences and they have influenced how you have evolved. Babies are often more competent than we give them credit for. They need milk, warmth and protection, but they also need to grow emotionally and socially, which begins to happen right from the start. The sense of self begins when development is at its earliest and the baby brain begins to organise information. How the brain organisation progresses is in direct relation to each baby's experience according to their internal and external worlds. Each baby is totally dependent on interactions with others to develop their sense of who they are; their self. They take in information and organise it into some sort of order, so it can make sense - this then becomes their internal working model [19].

Essential for survival, and right from birth, babies look for and are innately attuned to seek interactions with others. A baby in isolation cannot exist alone, they need 'an-other' for survival, which was a notion first introduced by a famous paediatrician and psychoanalyst, Dr Donald Winnicott who said, "There is no such thing as a baby ... if you set out to describe a baby, you will find you are describing a baby and someone. A baby cannot exist alone but is essentially part of a relationship" [20]. Babies are born with behaviours that ensure they have someone to care for them, for survival, these behaviors ensure close contact with the caregiver. Human babies are one of the most immature primates at birth. They cannot maintain their body temperature, reach their food source unaided, and are unable to regulate intense emotions; they depend on an-other for survival. Fussing or even crying, are all behaviours that trigger a parental response to provide care. As the baby matures so does their behavioural repertoire and behaviours such as smiling and cooing and reaching out become part of their communication [21]. Babies are not designed to be alone and if they are left alone, it can be a challenging experience for them.

Babies often struggle when they are separated for sleep. Some parents respond by cuddling their baby, others try some settling and others elect to be with their baby during sleep times. All these decisions are individual choices, and it is not for anyone else to judge. If parents elect to sleep separate to their baby, they may find that offering additional comforting at sleep time may assist the baby with the separation. Studies have shown that a baby sleeping within sensory range of their parent have natural and safe sleep [22]. Sensory range means within range of smelling, hearing and sensing their parents. This is especially so within the first months of life when the baby is vulnerable, yet developing so rapidly. Sensory range can be the baby sleeping in their own cot or bassinet nearby the parents, or it can also mean sharing the bed with their parents. There are a number of reputable organisations who have safe bedsharing and co-sleeping guidelines accessible for parents and professionals [23].

For years, research and studies have explored what helps a baby develop emotionally and socially so that a healthy, true sense of self that carries through to adulthood, can emerge. What it seems to boil down to is the quality of the relationship between the caregiver and the baby. This relationship or the interactional bond, serves as building blocks that buffer against adversity throughout life [21,24,25]. This bond literally shapes how the baby's brain grows. How this relationship looks is completely different to each individual situation, but it has some key characteristics. When observed from the outside, it is the interactions between individuals, the flow of energy that results in the two being in some sort of synchronous interplay. For example, the baby cries, the parent responds in a caring way and the baby calms. Or the parent tenses and the baby becomes alert and tense. Together the relationship works as one entity. This builds the baby's understanding of how relationships happen.

The parent noticing and responding to the baby's cues and interactions, allows the baby to grow to feel as if their experiences are real and worthy of recognition. This relationship becomes a deep and enduring bond that forms the foundations for the infant's understanding of what babies expect from interactions with others, right through into adulthood [26] [27]. That, in a nutshell, is how parents are the architects of the baby's brain, structurally, emotionally and socially for now and into the future.

Babies' brains are a work in progress at birth. They are pre-programmed to seek out their caregiver and learn, over time, to respond to comforting and soothing, all while the brain is still developing. At birth, babies are driven by primal brain functions such as breathing, sucking, swallowing and hunger. This brain also experiences emotions, but is unable as yet to make sense of them or to control the emotions because that requires access to more sophisticated brain functions than the baby initially has no access to [21,28]. So, in those moments when a parent feels overwhelmed, it is easy to slip into the mindset of the baby "giving me an hour's sleep" or "always doing this to me", as if there is some intent on the baby's part. That is certainly how it can feel, but in reality, all the baby is really doing is signaling you because they have a need which they cannot meet alone.

Over time, babies develop both emotionally and physically, but sometimes seeing them master physical tasks is easier than noticing the emotional growth. It is huge for a baby to coordinate input from the external world and to coordinate brain, muscles and all the nerves required to respond to what they are experiencing [28]. When you smile, your baby cannot respond with a smile initially, rather they may just stare, though in time, as their brain matures, they can respond with a smile and before you know it, there are also sounds that are in synchrony with your responses to them [29]. A beautifully coordinated, interactive event.

Next time you are with a three-month-old and they quietly 'coo', just stop and quietly coo back at them. In a little while, after the baby's brain has processed your response, you may hear another 'coo'. However if you miss it, or if you make a huge noise that frightens the baby, then that second and subsequent 'coo' may be less forthcoming. So the next time your baby cries, and you feel it is 'just crying' give yourself a moment to think that this is your baby telling you they have a need, in the best way they know how, without words. Babies' behavior is their language, so the more we watch and see, the more appropriately we can respond in a way that helps meet their needs in an appropriate way. This is the beginnings of you teaching your baby, through experience, what self-regulation is about [30,31]. Over the years, you will see your baby grapple with acquiring the skill of self-regulation. If you are tempted to rush expecting your baby to self-regulate and self soothe, remember there are days when we, as adults, do not have a grasp on self-calming ourselves. Keep in mind you need to be realistic about what we expect of growing babies.

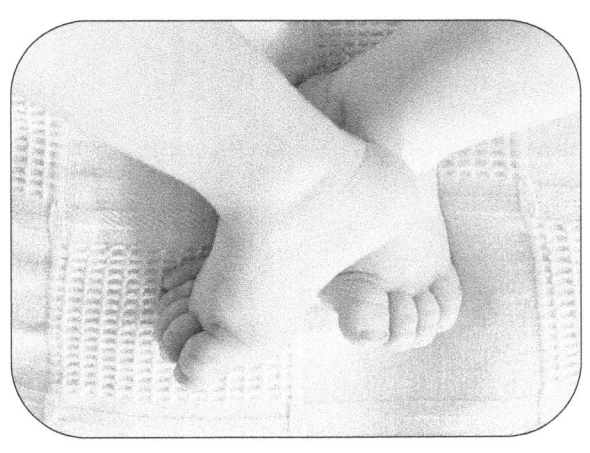

Chapter 3
Communication

Without words, babies need to rely on a range of ways to communicate [32]. An exercise I love doing with professionals is to ask them to communicate to a colleague that they are uncomfortable, without using speech, hands or body gestures. It is quite amusing and it tests the creativity of adults, so it is no wonder babies often struggle to communicate in a way that is clear to us. To indicate they are becoming unsettled, perhaps overwhelmed, babies start with what are called subtle cues; small actions to signal that not all is well. Perhaps they squirm, maybe they grimace or have a little furrow in their brow, or sometimes they just look away as if trying to stop whatever is overwhelming them from getting into their brain. They cannot say stop, help, I'm tired or you are jiggling me too much. All they can do is cue you. Being sensitive to those cues and behaviours can help parents tune into their baby.

Of course, there will be numerous cues we miss because they are far too subtle or we are focused elsewhere. If we miss them, they are most likely to become more obvious or what is called 'potent' [33]. A potent cue is hard to miss; squirming, grizzling, or even crying. There is no mistaking there is something wrong, but this is when parents can become overwhelmed by not knowing what is it that the baby needs. It seems impossible to be able to read every cue and clue to the internal world of the baby, but if you are aware that these subtleties exist, you will become an expert at reading your baby over time. Parents will become more and more able to decode their baby's communication, but it takes time and many mis-readings before the parent masters the art [34,35].

And, just when you think you read your baby really well, they develop more, and again you will adapt and grow with your baby.

Just remember that communication is a two-way street. As a parent you need to be clear about your communication as well as being receptive to the baby's [35]. Imagine if your baby is tired, and you are too, then your baby cries, you see them sucking their hand, and without another thought, you offer 'yet more' food. You may find your baby sucks enthusiastically to start with, but in no time, is lacking interest. Then they cry again. You find it really hard to hear your baby cry. In no time at all you are overwhelmed, even anxious or stressed because you don't know what else to do. It is enormous pressure that is compounded by the fact that babies are sensitive to their caregiver. Perhaps it's your stiffened body, or your less than snuggling hold, or perhaps you move faster or with more abrupt purpose. Whatever it is, your baby picks up on it and neither of you are able to respond calmly to each other.

This is such a common situation and one that results in much distress. Let's re-think that. Let's change one factor; your response. Your baby is hand sucking furiously, and you think, *I fed you an hour ago, you seemed to have fed really well, you've had lots and lots of wet and poo-ie nappies, so maybe you're not hungry, maybe you have a bubble of wind or maybe you just need a cuddle, and sucking your hands is a sign of discomfort this time rather than hunger.* You pick up your baby, cuddle and pat gently to help remove any wind ... the 'burp' is loud and clear, baby relaxes and you relax.

It can be enormously difficult to check in on your emotions when you are feeling the pressure, especially in the early days of parenting. However, even little tricks such as taking three long, slow, deep breaths can help you refocus on what is really happening in front of you rather than being swept away in the moment by rushed decisions and racing emotions. Each individual has learned ways throughout life to manage intense emotional responses. Yours might be breathing, or going for a jog. Well, jogging is not an option when your baby needs you, but it certainly is after your baby is in the care of another and you can go jogging to clear your head.

Sometimes even just naming the feeling; stop and think where you are feeling it and what is it you are feeling, may help. Anger, frustration, exasperation, sadness and helpless are just some words parents report they feel at those times. In the heat of the moment it is easy to overlook the baby's sensitivities, however, even raised voices can unsettle a baby. So, if you are a couple who resolve differences this way, just be sure you do it out of hearing range of your baby. As my mother used to say, *take it outside*. It is important to continue to resolve problems, but be aware that your default method may not be appropriate in range of the baby. You may need to work on finding your calm, be it a breath, walking away momentarily or putting on your favorite music. Whatever it is, practise it so it can drop into place when your baby needs you. Then you are less at risk of mismatching interactions with your baby because of your overwhelming feelings.

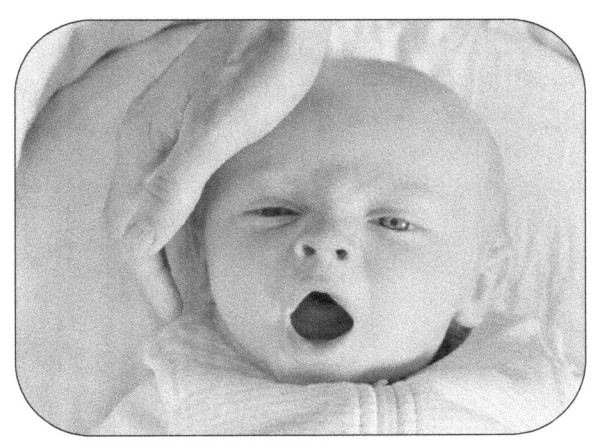

Chapter 4
Noah's family story

The story of mother Angelique, father Ben and baby Noah. (8 weeks)

"Noah is 8 weeks old and won't sleep in his cot, and never has"

This is how Angelique described their current situation.

"I am worried because he can only sleep in Ben's or my arms. He just screams when we put him down, he feeds and goes to sleep on my boob and only stays asleep while I cuddle or feed him. He seems to want to feed at least every 2 hours. He can stay awake for hours then cracks it. He has a lovely bassinet that he has never slept in. He can't sleep. He will sometimes sleep in the pram, but that's only sometimes. Is there something wrong with him, do you think? My mother says that he is hungry but our nurse says he is putting on weight and crying is normal for little babies. I've been told I should expect babies to cry, that's just what they do. So it must be me. What am I doing wrong? Ben is really helpful but he has gone back to work and I have to ask Mum to come over to help and she's getting really tired. She is starting to tell me he needs to learn to go to sleep. I know that, but how? All the other babies at my new parent's group sleep really well but some are bottle fed. Do you think I should offer him formula occasionally? I feel so bad that I can't work this out. I am trying things that people are telling me, but nothing is working. I think he could probably settle himself if I leave him for long enough, but I don't want to hear him screaming for that long. I am breast feeding and getting so tired that both Ben and my mum want me to get some help. I honestly don't know, my nurse talked to me about depression but I think I am just exhausted, actually I really don't know anymore. I am just really tired and I cry a lot, but that's what I do when I am really tired. Could it be hormones, maybe? I just don't know what to think anymore. I can't seem to get Noah in anything that looks like a routine. I have read so much and nothing seems to work. Is there anything you think you can do for us? Do you think maybe he has an allergy or intolerance or something, what about reflux? I am confused and I feel so useless as a mother. I love Noah and Ben is just great, but I am not enjoying this one little bit, and I can't believe I am actually even saying that, but it's true. Can you help us?"

There are 5 key things to think about here in relation to:
- Normal sleep, infant brains and relationship development
- Tired signs

- Calming Noah
- Family health
- Settling tips

Normal sleep, infant brains and relationship development

Noah is only 8 weeks old so he will have short and long sleeps and is still in what we call the 4th trimester. It is called this because human babies are born really immature, so much so they can't even regulate their temperature, nor get to their food source alone and they certainly can't regulate their emotions. So, they need lots of what you are already giving Noah; cuddles and care. When he is distressed he relies on you, or Ben or your mum to help him calm. If you leave him alone to sort himself out – he simply can't, because he doesn't have the brain capacity to do that. You are completely right in not wanting to leave him cry until he falls to sleep. Those are times when I consider the intuition of the mother, no matter how tired, remains strong, and as such you are protecting and caring for his welfare.

At 8 weeks of age I wouldn't expect to see a routine, so don't worry too much about that just for the moment. Noah will start to develop a sleep-feed-awake pattern, but realistically, that will shift and change from day to day at the moment. It will not be until around the end of the 3rd month that we might expect a baby to develop something that looks like a predictable routine. Even if patterns do develop early, they will change as your baby grows [36,37].

Just keep in mind, Noah has no idea he is even a separate person from you. All 'out there' in the world beyond him is more an experience or feeling, so there is nothing to tell him that he is ok when you are not with him. At this age, he is completely reliant on you to help him understand the world, including his own emotions and internal experiences. This time can be incredibly overwhelming for Noah as well, so he relies on the guidance from others to help him learn to even calm. Noah's relationship with you is unbelievably important for him now and for his future social and emotional development [38,39]. Sometimes in the business and stress of parenting, it is easy to forget this. So, make moments to just be with Noah, slow everything down and just 'be with' him. You don't have to do much, just let him explore you as you learn more about him. Watch him look for your face, watch him look away when he needs to process information, then watch him come back for more social interaction. You are his world and that link with you will help him be more able to calm and soothe when he is overwhelmed.

Tired signs

You will know when Noah is tired by watching for his tired signs that tell you his brain is preparing his body for sleep. Sometimes babies can be hard to read so be watchful for those signs around about an hour after he wakes from his last sleep. If he is awake much longer than that, he is at risk of becoming really overtired. Overtiredness in little babies can just look like they are awake and need some extra comforting to stay happy. Then, suddenly they start crying and need lots of help to calm. This is what happens when they are overtired, so the best time to help Noah drift to sleep is in that window of opportunity when he starts to look tired and before he is overtired.

Some of the early more subtle tired signs you would see in baby are:
- Paler face than usual
- A blank stare, glazed eyes
- Longer than usual blinks
- Motionless for short periods
- Red area near eyes or on brow line
- Furrowed brow

As tiredness increases, so do the cues and behaviours you may see:
- Spitting up small amounts of milk
- Grizzling for no obvious reason
- Yawning
- Jerking movements
- Face rubbing into your body
- Crying

Based on studies of infant sleep times, I would expect Noah would sleep anywhere from about half an hour, to 3-4 hours and occasionally he may have a 5 hour sleep, but that would not be common, if at all. For now, his tiny tummy needs frequent meals because it holds such a small volume. Frequent feeds are common so there will be many short sleeps allowing his tummy to be filled, he may stay awake a short while, and then go back to sleep. Even if you did offer formula to Noah it wouldn't guarantee he would sleep longer, in fact it may well cause him tummy discomfort. So if you can, hold back on that thought until we have talked more about sleep itself. As the months pass you will see more of a pattern emerge and you won't have to do anything to make it happen. The key is to watch for, and act on, those cues and behaviours so you know what to do next.

For now the most important things to remember are:
- In the first few months, babies have irregular sleep patterns
- A sleep pattern will develop eventually
- Sleep cues are your best friend, be watching for them
- Overtired babies struggle to sleep
- Don't worry too much at the moment about frequent feeding

Calming Noah

As already discussed, babies do not have access to the higher functioning parts of the brain necessary for self-soothing. So, when Noah is distressed, he needs you to help him calm. He won't need you forever, but for now he is reliant on you to help him calm. He just can't do it himself, no matter what you read or what you are told. Babies this age need an adult to help them learn to calm [40].

When Noah cries, even though sometimes it can feel like so much pressure, just remember that Noah is not wanting or trying to do this. He is just expressing he has a need and he needs someone to help him with it. Some really basic things can help babies, however, there is one really difficult thing - babies rely on us to calm them. If, as adults, we are feeling agitated, anxious or frustrated, our body tells our baby this. We become rigid or we tend to jiggle rather than gently sway and pat calmly. We are also inclined to be a bit louder and more frantic with our patting and shhing. For a moment, just imagine what it must be like as a baby relying on another to help them, and they are offered this abrupt and often not gentle form of comforting. Sadly, the baby won't settle, and nor will you, and around in an unhappy circle you can go.

Your baby needs to feel connected to someone to help them regulate strong emotions. It can be easy to interpret your baby's cries and fussing as annoying. Try to monitor your own emotions, and if needed and possible, allow your partner or mother to do some of the comforting, while you have a break.

The same applies to Ben and your mother when they are feeling stressed or anxious. They too should be able to allow you and each other to comfort Noah. When Noah shows tired signs, you may need to take him to a calm environment if he is unable to wind down. However, only do that if he is unable to calm, because depending on his temperament and his level of tiredness, he may be able to calm even though he is not in a darkened, quiet room. Some babies with easy going temperaments often drift to sleep more readily, despite the environmental stimulation. Some babies are more wired and alert and can't wind down without help. Just monitor him to see where he calms most easily and keep that in mind for times when he is struggling. Just a note on calming, if you use the pram and are tempted to put a cover over the pram to keep out the stimulation, be sure the cover is not of thick material, and that it doesn't cover the entire pram. Air must be able to flow easily through and around, so use a light fabric and cover only half of the open area so air movement is not restricted.

Another thing that helps many babies sleep is being swaddled or wrapped. This provides a sense of being snuggled in and being held, but also helps minimise the sleep disruptions that occur with the 'startle reflex'. When a baby's sensors are stimulated, particularly suddenly by a noise, a movement, or even their own hiccup, then their startle reflex is activated. What we see is baby flinging their arms up and out, fingers splayed, and then they recoil into a fetal position. Nothing can stop that reflex, but a wrap or swaddle can minimise the chance of it waking the baby.

A note of caution though; there are safety issues to consider. Make sure it is not restrictive across the baby's chest, and that the hips can flop outwards as the baby sleeps. Also, if using a wrap, ensure it is well secured so the fabric cannot drape up and over the baby's face. If using a wearable swaddle or sleeping bag, allow the arms to flex up into a natural position across the chest but also ensure the neck opening will not allow the baby's head to slip down into the sleep swaddle. Babies also overheat very easily because they don't have a mature, self-cooling mechanism, so ensure babies always sleep with their head uncovered and not bundled in multiple blankets. The rule of thumb is normally, one layer more than what you would have on; perhaps a singlet, then a onesie, sleeping sack or swaddle and if really cold, one light blanket. Remember that once your baby begins to roll you need to be sure they have their arms free.

When your baby sleeps is critical. The actual hours on the clock are not as important as getting the timing right for Noah. To know when it is the right time, will be when his tired signs indicate he is ready for sleep. If you try to get him to sleep according to the clock, you will find he may not be tired and ready for sleep at the 'prescribed' sleep time, and this can cause a lot of distress. Trying to make a baby sleep when they are not tired is not going to end well at all. Distress will reign, so just follow his lead and calm him in preparation for sleep by rocking him in your arms and placing him into his bassinet when he is drowsy. That way he can experience his cot at sleep time, while he is calm. Should he begin to cry just follow the settling steps below.

Family health

Caring for an unsettled baby can be relentless, exhausting and often not very rewarding, so you need to have ways to break the cycle if you start to spiral into distress. Long, slow, deep breaths have been shown to change the electrical activity in the brain. It can change from highly charged and what looks like over-aroused to slower, calmer patterns.

It is not a weakness to ask for help; rather I consider it a strength and a sign of your own emotional maturity. Maybe, pop baby into the pram and go for a walk in the garden or use the baby carrier and go for a walk. Help you to help yourself to notice and try to bring yourself down to calm, so you will be more able to be emotionally available for Noah. Yes it is hard sometimes, but worth building the skill, because as a parent you will need it in the future anyway!

It is hard to be supportive of each other when both parents are feeling the strain of an unsettled child. Keep in mind, if you can do as much as you can together, you will both benefit, and so will your baby. Both of you are parents and responsible for Noah's care, so sharing is important for you and for Noah. If you are still struggling emotionally once there are longer and less stressful sleep times in your family, I strongly suggest you chat with your Doctor or Maternal Child and Family Health Nurse, because there are a range of helpful resources out there they can guide you to. Please also keep in mind, that ongoing stress can result in anxiety and even depression for both parents. If either of you are finding this challenging time relentless, it is best to look for help early in yours and Noah's life.

Actual settling tips:

Keeping in mind babies drift to sleep more readily when they are calm:

- Babies can't self-calm, so they need your help
- You need to offer experiences that help your baby calm when they show tired signs
- Take notice of how your baby responds to your comforting efforts

If one form of comforting is not working after about 15 seconds, then move to another:

- When Noah shows tired signs, reduce the external stimulation so he can start to wind down for sleep
- Not all babies need a quiet dark room to sleep, but if Noah is struggling to calm, take him somewhere quiet where the lighting is dulled
- Change his nappy and pop him into his wrap or swaddle
- Cuddle him until he is calm, but not quite asleep
- Place him into his bassinet
- Gently rest your hands across his body to provide a sense of you being there
- Quietly shh shh and calmly and gently rock his body ever so slightly if he is beginning to squirm or grizzle
- If he cries he might respond to you patting the

- side of his hip and upper leg area
- Take notice to see what Noah finds calming
- He may just like you gently holding one of your hands over his body to comfort him, and with the other hand you could gently pat the mattress near his feet
- If he is not calming, try singing. It's a very powerful way to engage other parts of the brain that are not involved in the distress
- If Noah remains upset and is not calming to any of the above, pick him up and cuddle him until he calms
- Once calm, try him again in his cot

Don't expect Noah to go to sleep immediately the first time you try this. You need to do it two or three times before each sleep and if he can't settle, then cuddle or feed him to sleep, and just try again next time. This is all about offering Noah experiences that are not stressful, so that he can begin to calm and to experience what calm is. If you try this at each sleep, it allows Noah to experience it repeatedly so that he begins to anticipate your comforting. Be realistic and don't expect him to understand immediately.

After trying the above for three days and nights this was the feedback from Angelique and Ben:

"It's unbelievable! He's like a new baby. He sleeps mostly in his bassinet and it takes hardly any effort to comfort him, and he's even gone off to sleep from awake without me doing anything except sitting beside him a couple of times. I can't believe we are saying this and I fear our magic bubble might burst, but he's so happy to go to sleep now.

You asked me what I thought were the pivotal moments for the change.

- I think I started thinking about what it must be like for him, a bit more
- I stopped trying to make him go to sleep
- I watched for his tired signs and we are sure now that he was staying awake too long between sleeps
- I can see now that when we were working hard to calm him we weren't really watching him to see what worked, we were watching for sleep only. We can now see what he actually likes and what makes him more upset. He loves me stroking his forehead and he just calms and goes all relaxed.
- We still sometimes cuddle him to sleep because we love to, but we know to also let him sleep in his bassinet as well. It has been really nice to know we can enjoy cuddling him to sleep rather than always feeling guilty. It's just so nice sometimes.
- We talked about this and think the most important thing is us understanding more about Noah and how to give him love instead of just expect him to do what we thought babies should do, and how we thought he *should* sleep.
- We sincerely hope this helps others in a similar situation because we would never wish what we had onto anyone if it could be avoided.

My reflections

There was nothing in this story that was rocket science. These parents are good at being parents. They were doing all they could with the understanding they had, and most of all, they knew to ask for help when they were struggling.

Update:

"Noah is great! He's 12 weeks old and we just thought you might like to know, he has never looked back and neither have we. He 'talks' all the time, smiles and is now sleeping for 3 to 4 hours at a time at night, and in the morning, he has a huge sleep, sometimes 2 ½ hours, and then occasionally he has another long one during the day, though the others are more often short. But we don't care and he doesn't care. He is growing like a mushroom and my mum wants to pass on her thanks and to say she wished she had known all of this when she had me! Tell other parents that it really can get so much better if you get the right sort of help."

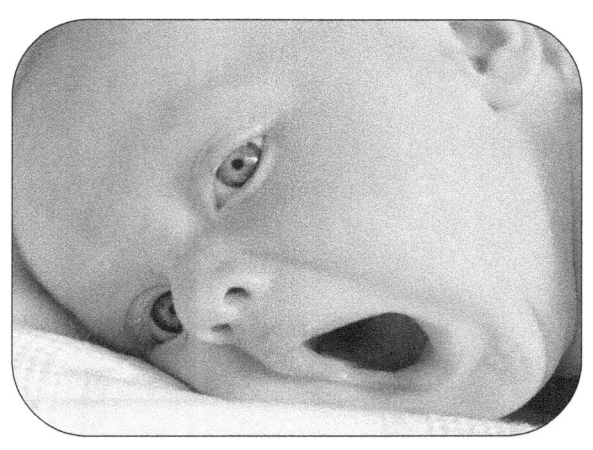

Chapter 5
Avi's family story

The story of mother Nicola, father Josh and baby Avi (19 weeks)

"Avi's sleep is a disaster since her 4 month sleep regression"

This is how Nicola described their current situation.

"My baby Avi is 19 weeks and sleep has become a disaster. She slept so well until she turned 4 months old and for the last 3 weeks she has woken and screamed at every sleep. It's just getting worse, not better. My doctor and nurse tell me it's normal sleep regression. She is not sick either. So how do I stop it? She is putting on weight but we are so so tired. My partner travels a lot so I do it all at night but even the day sleeps have gone crazy so I don't get any downtime at all now. Avi used to sleep for at least 2 hours twice a day and even three times some days, and have at least one or two naps and that was my saviour, but it's all gone now. Bed time is around 7pm after her bath and book time. Now she needs to be cuddled to sleep and then only sleeps for 20 to 40 minutes. Now it is taking up to an hour to get her to sleep. **I have recently been putting her in my bed, but even though she sleeps, I don't, aghhhhh.** All I do all day and night is think about her sleep. She feeds well, I do breast and bottle, and feeding has never been an issue, but she wants breastfeeds all the time now. I just don't know how to get back to where we were when she would sleep through with maybe one feed. She used to drift to sleep in the lounge room, and that is just not happening any more. Avi has a 2 year old sister and Avi is now waking her at night and I feel like our world is now revolving around Avi's sleep. I just can't be spending hours getting Avi to sleep while I've got a 2 year old running around, as she is getting really needy now. I know she needs more attention, but it's getting impossible for us all. Seriously, I don't know what to do. I just want to cry and I feel like I am living in a **delirious** fog. Now we all have yet another cold which is just great. We are one very unhappy house and no matter what I do I can't get Avi back to her old sleep routine. I keep trying to stick to times but it's been a disaster. I've tried rocking her to sleep and feeding her to sleep, but that takes hours and I am so afraid of spoiling her and I know I will be creating a rod for my own back. So I tried letting her cry, not for long, just 10 minutes or so to see if she will sleep, but not even that is working. I try everything for 5 to 10 minutes because I know that gives her a chance to understand, but it's just not working, nothing is working. It doesn't matter how I get her to sleep, she wakes again in no time. I didn't have trouble with sleep regression with my other daughter and feel completely at a loss. I really am over it all and don't know how much longer we can keep going like this."

There are some key things to think about here:
- Sleep regression
- Overtiredness
- Brain development
- Spoiling babies
- Settling tips

Sleep regression

Because of their enormous growth rate, especially in the first 3 years, babies are constantly changing. Just when you think you understand what's happening, it changes again. Sleep is no exception. In those first few months the baby is working very hard on making meaning of every experience. We often take for granted our world around us, but to babies it is all new. Making meaning of interactions and experiences is how they grow to understand. What makes the brain process information is often related to repetition. A one-off experience is unlikely to have huge impact, unless it is catastrophic. Rather, experiences over and over ensure the neural connections associated with that experience are strengthened until they become strong, fast neural pathways [40]. I often describe this as being like when you walk through the long grass and you leave footprints, but the more you walk along that same path, the more defined the path becomes. In no time, the tramped down grass becomes a clear, accessible and easy to navigate pathway. Similar to that of a neural pathway, the more it is activated and the nerve messages are sent along a particular route, the stronger the pathway becomes. Repeated sequences of nerve activation help to make experiences and interactions predictable [40].

The growing brain develops in a particular sequential way, so when one part of the brain is well developed it becomes the building block for the next expansion of brain growth. For example, for a baby to be able to roll over, coordination of the head, shoulders and body muscle movement needs to occur. It is only with the development of these necessary individual components, including brain wiring, that the baby is able to actually roll. What is often seen is that one part of the development or system will go on hold, or become irregular, while another is working on developing.

So, when a baby reaches around 4 months of age there is already a complex brain network of neural activity happening. But then comes a huge shift in capacity; for the first time the baby can clearly visually focus on distance, so the world suddenly becomes much bigger and more interesting. Simultaneously, voluntary and purposeful movement comes to the fore. For the first time, the baby can actually reach out and make the world around them respond. The toys on the play gym can now be touched and tapped so they tinkle and shine. The baby can intentionally move them after much concentration and effort so they can make the toys respond by their own actions. That alone is an enormous achievement. Your once smiling baby can now show full-bodied excitement when they see you. No longer is it just a smile; it is arms, legs and face, all alive and telling you how thrilled they are to see you. And those eyes, you can't look away from them when a four month old tells you it is time to talk, and talk they do. The vocalisations suddenly seem robust, expressive and intense. And guess what happens when all this development is bursting into bloom? Sleep changes, and often not in a good way.

This is what is often called sleep regression, but really it is just sleep changing as the body, brain and mind progress in huge leaps. So it could be thought of in terms of sleep progression, as baby is moving to a new and higher level of development. We call it regression because babies begin to have changed sleep and social patterns, but really it is all part of the huge leap to a more organised, integrated, higher functioning brain and body coordinated system. This is really a time to delight in the amazing development shifts being made, rather than fear and worry about sleep disturbances and how disruptive they can be for the family.

However, this is very easy to say when you are not the one managing on half, if even that much sleep. When the entire family is disrupted and sleep deprived and now catching every cough and cold that is around because the immune system is compromised because of sleep disturbances; that is really hard work.

What a baby needs during the phase of interrupted sleep, is understanding and kind, compassionate care giving. It is impossible to imagine how disruptive the processes must be for a baby going through such a monumental internal growth spurt, however, we do know what we can do to help at this time. This means reaching deep into that parenting well and pulling out as much kindness, calm and compassion you can. To help this it can be good to keep in mind … that this is but a phase, and not a life sentence. Like all phases, this too shall pass. Your baby needs comforting when distressed so she learns that with distress comes calm. She doesn't quite know how it happens but repeated comforting when she is unsettled means she will then be more adapted to calming herself when distressed.

A good description is to call it co-regulating, or co-piloting. As you show her calm can happen, eventually she begins to become less overwhelmed with the understanding that calm will happen. Babies rely heavily on their parents to be able to help them through times of disruption because they just can't do it themselves [38]. Comforting when distressed and plenty of talking together, smiling and little games that encourage you to take turns at interaction are great. Let your baby lead the interactions because this too helps the brain process interaction and communication. These are times when we can really see that the power of the parent in just being with a baby is, in itself, a means of keeping calm [41].

When your baby is passing through the phase, resist the urge to sleep train, or to leave your baby to cry until they work it out for themselves, as this may actually compound the distress rather than help them progress through this stage. This is definitely not the time to try to get the sleep patterns you dream of in place. That will all happen in time. For now, comfort and pay homage to the enormous internal shifts that are occurring in your baby so you can offer the kindest and most timely and appropriate care, despite your delirium. Once you can embrace this transition phase, you will probably be more able to calm yourself so you can in turn, calm your baby.

Overtiredness

I would consider overtiredness to almost be the number one enemy of baby sleep. Think about this from an adult perspective. How are you when you are overtired? A bit sensitive, maybe even grumpy? How well do you settle for sleep when you are deliriously tired but don't get to bed? And when you finally do, perhaps your eyes are wide open and you are solving the world problems; then sleep becomes elusive. Yes, that's overtired. Anyone with a toddler knows that life reaches its most challenging peak when a toddler becomes overtired. Babies too, need so much more support to get off to sleep when their brain has reached that chaotic state of overtiredness. If overtired then calming in preparation for sleep is much harder to achieve, and overtired is often the melting point for many families. When a baby is not sleeping well, we often miss the ever-important tired signs, because everyone is tired and subtle unfocussed stares, the momentary long blinks, seem to be happening all the time.

If you are living in an overtired world, make every effort to watch for and act on tired signs, because that can make an enormous difference to a baby's ability to settle, or not, for sleep. Overtired babies are far more difficult to care for.

Another thing happens when the entire family is tired and overwhelmed; it is that there are often mismatches in communication, which in turn lead to increasing emotional arousal and even more mismatches [41]. For example, a grizzling baby who is tired and ready for sleep, may be interpreted to be just fussing and so a parent may try shaking some jingly toys to create a diversion. For the moment, that quietens the baby but in no time at all baby is screaming and no one knows why. So then we need to start looking for causes. The cause has come and gone. The baby was tired and needed additional calming and preparation for sleep, but tired parents can miss this and accidently overstimulate a baby who is already on the edge. The result is a family of unhappiness and distress because cues were misread.

'Spoiling' Babies

Babies need care, by responding to and caring for them you are not spoiling them. That is a fact. They need the care from an adult who can see they have a need and who can respond by offering appropriate care for that need, which is much easier said than done. It is called responsive or contingent care. That is, it is care based on what the baby needs [42]. Babies, however, can be really hard to read, which can make the parents' job of offering appropriate care, even harder. If you don't offer your baby care when they signal they need it, they will not be able to manage themselves, and if left for extended periods at sleep time, they can become overwhelmed by the experience and they become flooded with stress hormones. This has been seen in babies as young as 4 months old when undergoing controlled crying interventions. Although they did seem to be quieter for longer periods of time, thought to be asleep, they continued to have elevated stress hormones circulating in their bodies [11]. You are not at risk of spoiling a baby by helping them manage intense emotional distress, you are supporting them by being the circuit breaker of the stress until they learn to do that for themselves. At 4 months of age babies are certainly not capable of internal regulation of their stress response system once it's activated, so they need help. This is just not spoiling.

Perhaps the idea of spoiling originates from when parents are struggling to see what their baby is cueing, and perhaps they don't place them into their cot when calm, for fear of them waking. In this case the baby becomes accustomed to only experiencing sleep in the parents arms, and therefore begins to expect that. If a parent is able to read and respond to the cues, then is likely to feel more confident to place the baby into their sleep place at sleep time, and comfort them as needed. This allows the baby to experience comforting while in the cot but still have access to cuddles if unable to settle. Fear of 'what if' can distract parents from the here and now and may result in parenting in a fixed manner, rather than being guided by the baby's cues and behaviours. Again, this is easier said than done when parenting through the haze of exhaustion.

To compound the fog that gets in between what we feel and what we see, is the fact that we all come to parenting with different experiences and sometimes a baby can actually trigger some of the parents' own childhood experiences. This is often seen when a baby cries and rather than the parent softening into just carrying them or cuddling to calm and allowing the baby to calm, the parent can become intense and insistent on stopping the fussing or crying rather than pausing to attempt to offer a calming experience to the baby. The result can be a more distressed baby and parent. The past can trigger feelings that are not directly related to the baby in your arms, here and now, but perhaps you find yourself thinking about how you were parented and some of your early experiences. These thoughts can filter into your here and now and somehow mask what is actually happening. You are then responding to the thoughts of your past and perhaps not of your baby in this very moment. This is a completely normal phenomenon that occurs in early parenthood, that basically come from the parents' childhoods that infuses into the current situation. Sometimes these can be helpful thoughts and memories [43] or they can have the potential to interfere with how the parent sees and cares for the baby in front of them [44]. It is sometimes helpful to be aware of what you are thinking when you respond to your baby. Your thought processes are often very normal, but be conscious of how these may be influencing what you do and how you offer your baby care, especially at sleep time, when everyone is more highly sensitive.

Settling tips

What Avi needs is for you to help her to calm when her central nervous system becomes over-aroused. She can't just take a big long calming breath like we can, so leaving her to cry will not help her learn to calm and drift to sleep.

A kind predictable pattern of calming will help Avi prepare for sleep:

- Cuddles, rocking, and or singing quietly in her darkened room is a great start
- When she cries, comfort her, start by comforting her in her cot if you like, but if that is not calming her, then pick her up, calm her and then pop her back in her cot
- Try to have a predictable set of calming steps in your mind so Avi experiences them over and over so then she can begin to anticipate them, and ultimately respond by calming
- Try not to plan her sleeps by the clock, rather watch her body. If she looks tired it is the ideal time for sleep, even if she just woke 40 minutes before. Eventually she will lengthen out the time between sleeps, as she gets more sleep
- When she wakes after 20 to 40 minutes, offer her comforting in her cot, just for a short time, to see if you can lull her back to sleep. Even a little cuddle might do the job, then place her back in her cot. Avoid persisting for long periods because she has just had a powernap and may resist resettling for

quite some time, so don't persist for long periods at all

- Comforting in her cot with shhing or mattress patting or singing, allows Avi to experience something between waking and feeding, to help guide her understanding of returning to sleep when she wakes after 30 to 40 minutes or less. This waking represents the end of one sleep cycle and your calming is an effort to encourage her into her next sleep cycle. BUT if she can't drift to sleep in a minute or so, don't persist if she is distressed, just pick her up and watch for her next tired signs, then settle her again for sleep

- You might want to put a chair beside the cot so you can be comfortable and more patient as she drifts to, and back to sleep

- When going to sleep or resettling Avi, keep settling times really short, because long struggles won't benefit anyone. If she is not calming to your comforting efforts, then just cuddle her and try again, but if she isn't calming or if you feel over it all, just cuddle or feed her to sleep and start again next time

- After a few days and nights, when Avi has experienced your comforting each time, she will begin to internalise the pattern you are creating, and will more likely be able to calm when you respond to her

- As you have noted, babies who once used to sleep happily amongst the household sounds, can also shift to being aware and alert to any noise and you end up tippy-toeing around. If that is the case, it seems like her increased social awareness

now means she needs to sleep somewhere a little less stimulating, it might be time to go to her own room for day sleeps if she is alerting to her world around her at sleep time
- For the moment, focus less on the clock and more on what Avi is telling you. When she is looking tired, then that is sleep time, when she can't settle, just cuddle her, without referring to clock times for a few days at least and watch how sleep progresses
- Even though Avi might have been able to feed once only overnight, that will inevitably shift through this progression. Don't try to force that pattern back. It will come back if you offer her comforting now, even if it means extra feeds overnight for a couple more weeks. Just remember to fit in only a minute or two of trying to calm her before each feed so she experiences that each time, it gives her the opportunity to settle back to sleep if she's not hungry
- Her increased mobility at this time isn't very helpful right now, however be sure Avi is in a sleeping bag where she can have her arms free, once she starts to roll. This is really important for safety reasons as well as for developing her own autonomy
- If Avi has moved around the cot, try to resist the urge to reposition her back in the middle. The middle just doesn't matter to her, and if you lift her to reposition her, she may well expect to be lifted up, and the disappointment that follows will be expressed most probably in an enormous cry, first by her and then by you!

- It doesn't sound like Avi sleeping in with you is your plan, but keep in mind if you are super tired and you lay in your bed to feed her, you will most likely drift to sleep. So, plan in advance, try to make your bed a safe co-sleeping environment so even the unplanned sleeps together are planned and therefore the SIDS risk is reduced [45]. That way you might both sleep a little better too. This is also a good time to remind you that there are evidenced based recommendations and guidelines that help parents provide a safe sleeping environment that include sleeping your baby on her back, making sure bedding cannot cover her face or overheat her, that she needs to sleep in a smoke free environment and that there are things we can do to minimise the risk of sudden infant death events [46].

My reflection

This is a disruptive phase for everyone, but remaining kind and trying to think about what might be happening during this growth phase, will help you provide the care that Avi needs right now. Don't focus too much on getting back to where you were. This is more about experiences in the here and now that help Avi feel more able to calm. Then your once loved pattern has a better chance of returning. Avoid the pressure to look for a quick fix in the form of sleep training, because in this amazing growth phase, that may cause more disruption than calm. Gentle care that is shaped around Avi's cues and behaviours is more likely to restore calm to your home.

Also for your 2 year old there is plenty of information about toddlers and new babies that you may find very helpful.

You are by no means the only parent in this situation and some ideas for toddlers are great to guide the very tired parents of two ... or more! Parents' feedback is that the website articles are helpful [47], but have a look around to see what works best for your family.

The length of time this sleep regression period lasts is variable and the level of impact can be influenced by many things, one significant one being how you respond. If you help your baby calm, she is more likely to come through in a happier way than if you try to force her into a pattern that may involve long periods of distress for you all.

Update

"As you asked, I am getting back to you now 3 weeks since your advice. It made so much sense and it felt so much nicer to be able to offer Avi love rather than 'tough love', which I had been strongly advised to do by many people. I am so glad I didn't bend to that pressure. I now do a little rock of Avi sometimes to help her settle down, or I just pat her bottom. She is rolling now, so I don't move her anymore into the middle, I just settle her in wherever she is. That sounds like so little but it has actually made it easier. That really sad crying has stopped. She hasn't done those awful screaming cries since we started this so it is so much calmer in our home now. Occasionally, I do still need to pick her up for cuddles but now I feel good about that too. It was such a relief when I let go of trying to get the routine back. I watch her more now and I know I was definitely letting her get too tired and then she would lose the plot completely. She woke twice last night and as I always do now, I did some settling moves first. It's pretty short because she is still congested a bit and I think the feed helps her clear it so she can sleep. Her day sleeps are miraculously almost back to what they were. I wouldn't have believed it if I hadn't lived through this, but I think all Avi needed was more love and less pressure from me for a routine while she was going through her sleep changes. I felt really panicked though because I thought it was going to keep getting worse. It really has been so good for us to see how we need to watch her and be guided by her, and to think more about us as a family and her experiences. And we are thinking more about what she needs from us to help her calm. With a toddler, I feel like I am in a rush all the time and I think I was getting stressed and even more rigid thinking that a routine was the only way to keep us all happy. But really, we are all much happier now and a kind of routine has somehow made its way back without me worrying too much.

You asked me what I thought really made the difference. I think all of the above, but mostly our understanding that Avi is growing and developing and that there are times she will be unhappy, and if I respect those times and comfort her when she needs me, then somehow it will all work out. She needs us more than I really thought she did, but not in a bad way, in a normal baby way. I am sleeping now and the family is happy and almost all healthy again. And I know this was not specifically about her 2 year old sister, but she is also so much calmer now that I am being kinder to everyone in the house. Because I am less tired and frustrated I can see when she is more likely to lose the plot and I am getting in earlier. We are all in a much better place."

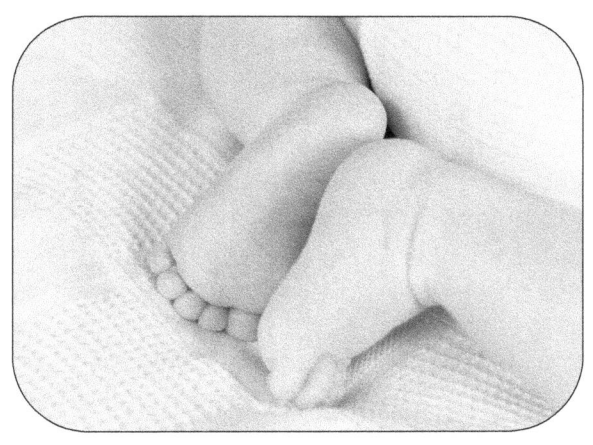

Chapter 6
Ayaz's family story

The story of mother Ayla, father Ceren and baby Ayaz (8 months)

"Ayaz wakes 10 or more times a night for a feed"

"Ayaz feeds a lot through the night. The feed is quick thankfully, and he falls straight back to sleep but I am 8 weeks pregnant and very tired. I don't think he needs this much milk and he is growing very well. He is 9.4kg but is wanting lots of milk through the night still. He goes to sleep easily, I just feed him and put him in the cot and he stays asleep. I want to start bottles but he will not drink my milk from a bottle. I am going back to work next month for a little while. I try to give him more food but he only eats a little bit of food and then he shuts his mouth and turns away and won't let me put the spoon near him. I think he is not hungry for food, only milk.

When he wakes at night I feed him because he cries very loudly if I do not feed him and he is too big now for me to rock to sleep anymore. He is clingier than ever and now my husband can only rock him to sleep sometimes, but I still have to feed him at least 3 or 4 times when he cannot get him to stop crying. He cries a lot if I do not feed him. I am very tired and would like to stop feeding so much at night and to get him on the bottle. He sleeps well during the day but overnight he does not sleep well at all. Can you help him sleep longer at night?"

There are some key things to think about here:
- Sleep associations
- Sleep cycles
- Separation anxiety
- Starting bottles
- Dream feeding
- Settling tips

Sleep associations

It sounds incredibly tiring for you right now, and perhaps Ayaz has grown to think the only way to go to sleep is comfort sucking at your breast. So, let's talk about that first.

Babies learn to expect what going to sleep 'looks like'. They know what to expect and anticipate each part of the process based on what they have experienced. Babies make it particularly clear that they know what to expect, especially if you try to change the order or way they go off to sleep. These expectations are called 'sleep associations' because they are what your baby associates with going to sleep.

In Ayaz's case it seems that he is reliant on the breast for sleep. So each time he wakes, and the breast is not available, then he does not know how to return to sleep. Babies who comfort suck to sleep are usually babies who have never had a dummy or pacifier because they already have the breast, so the sucking is often more about comforting rather than actively feeding. For some babies, feeding off to sleep works, and it works for their family, but it sounds like it has become difficult for you now with so many wakings.

So, the tips (on the next page) will include how to move away from the associations where you have to be with him every time he goes to sleep. There are some sleep associations that are good though. I call them independent sleep associations, which are the things that your baby associates with sleep time, but are independent of you. Things like background noise; such as white or pink noise, is completely harmless and just quietly happens in the background during the entire sleep time. It means you are not directly needed for the sleep message to be happening. Things like a sleeping bag and a darkened room also can be helpful independent sleep associations. Don't be afraid of independent sleep associations at all. It is the ones that depend on you being needed to get sleep happening that are the ones that can be tiring and may prevent babies from finding their own way to sleep. In the tips further below I will talk about addressing that a little more.

Sleep cycles

Another thing that is linked with frequent waking is the actual architecture of baby sleep. Babies have sleep cycles just like adults do, except they are much shorter than adults' - about half the length - and the time spent in each phase within the cycle is different to adult sleep. However, they do have a start, middle and end of a cycle. In a perfect world when a baby ends one sleep cycle, which lasts around 45 minutes, they can just drift back into another sleep cycle. We know that this has happened because the baby has been asleep for an hour and a half or more, because one sleep cycle is about 45 minutes, so two sleep cycles have been linked together when the baby sleeps longer periods [48]. This linking of the sleep cycles is often the time when babies struggle if they have grown accustomed to doing something, like using comfort sucking to go to sleep. These babies stir at the end of the first sleep cycle, and rather than just squirming around a little and going back into another sleep cycle, they need whatever it is they usually need to go back off to sleep. So, if the breast is not available they will call out because that is how they know sleep happens. For that reason, I would like you to start feeding Ayaz until he is very nearly asleep, then, remove your breast from his mouth. If needed, cuddle him for a little longer to get him to sleep, then place him into his cot.

Over the following week, try to finish the sucking time when he is less drowsy, so eventually you will be removing the breast when he finishes the nutritious, enthusiastic sucking. Also as the days pass, try to cuddle him after a feed until he is a tiny bit less sleepy each time, so he is increasingly aware that he is going into his cot. This will help move towards him drifting to sleep without your breast in his mouth, as well as also allowing him to experience going into his cot awake. But don't rush this because adjustment takes time with babies, and it will be more tolerable for Ayaz if it is a progressive change. Remember to keep moving forward with the change, little by little, so you don't get stuck in one stage. This experience will then help Ayaz to be more able to drift into a second sleep cycle without relying on you.

Separation anxiety

I suspect I am right in thinking Ayaz has had his current sleep patterns for a while, perhaps not waking as often, but waking multiple times overnight and needing you to help him back to sleep. What we have to also think about now is that babies go through what is called 'separation anxiety'. This phase starts anywhere around 6 to 7 months and lasts until around 9 months. The importance of thinking about this is because your baby now knows that he is all alone when you are not with him. He will know to look for you and call out for you [49]. It is also a time when babies may respond less to their other parent, and when they were once able to calm for sleep by being comforted, for example by Dad, they now reject Dad and keep calling until Mum comes, or it may happen that they keep calling until Dad comes. With this new understanding, Ayaz finds being separated from you really challenging, so becomes, what parents often describe, as 'clingy'. But really what he is doing is adjusting to this new concept of you still existing when he cannot see you, which causes some babies to be more prone to distress when being left alone, and without you. Babies have been separated from the parent before this age, however this is a new awareness of you being somewhere else when you are gone from them. They now know they are really alone; so, they hold on tight at times of impending separation.

It is a phase and it will pass if you are thoughtful about your baby's experience and how hard it is for them to separate. If you focus on making separations as small, and as tolerable for your baby as possible, then he will progressively learn that the separation poses no real threat to his existence, because you always return. But for now, Ayaz doesn't have the confidence that he will be okay without you, so he may have trouble separating. It will help him adjust if you remain kind and offer him care in a predictable way so he can begin to trust the process. During this time, if he really doesn't want to be alone, then don't force him. Reassure him and keep separations brief so he grows to learn that you will return. This helps him through this phase which is more likely to result in him watching you leave the room without him becoming hysterical.

Starting bottles

Ayaz sounds like he knows his mind and he is not interested in milk from a form that is anything less than you. You have a couple of options. He is old enough to not need his milk from a bottle, so if he is not interested, then offer him milk in a sippy cup. It is good to offer him milk in either a bottle or cup in a way that is not similar to breast feeds, so it is clear you are not trying to offer a substitute breast feed. Offer him milk while in his high chair, or sit him up on your knee so he is less in a breast feeding position. Don't bother trying to trick him, because babies are smart and laying him in a breast feeding position and then offering a bottle may be something he completely rejects. If you really want him to have a bottle, then allow him to become familiar with it; letting him examine the bottle more, touch, feel, play with it, and you may find he even puts it to his own mouth. This increased control often helps babies accept the idea of a bottle.

Also, just allow him to have small amounts of either your milk or formula in the bottle, so you don't feel he has to drink the entire lot just yet. Little by little he can adjust, if you don't force him. Just try to respect the fact that it is not what he is accustomed to and may need some adjustment time through gentle exploration of the bottle before he is interested in drinking it. Also, when Ayaz is feeding less overnight you will probably notice he will feed because he is hungry, rather than just for comfort. This is when Ayaz may become more interested in the bottle. With reduced overnight feeding you are bound to see an increase in his interest in food. Then you can start to increase his dairy intake in the form of cheese and yoghurt for example, and that will take some pressure off him drinking his daily milk requirements, especially if he is not thrilled by the idea of the bottle or cup. For now, go gently and allow Ayaz time to explore the idea of a bottle or sippy cup and even if you do feel desperate, resist the urge to insisting on him drinking, because he may well object and shut his mouth very firmly. If that happens, there will be absolutely no chance of him drinking from the bottle or cup if he chooses to keep his mouth shut.

Dream feed

The following tips focus on encouraging you to not offer Ayaz your breast immediately every waking time overnight. Sometimes though, we worry that our babies may be hungry when they wake overnight, so to help with that perhaps you could offer him a feed before you go to bed. This is called a 'dream feed' because you don't wait for Ayaz to ask for the feed, but rather you pick him up, while he is asleep, offer a nice big feed, and pop him back in his cot. It is done with the lights low, no social interaction and not even a nappy change. Just up, feed and back to the cot. That way you know when Ayaz next wakes he is probably not hungry and you will feel more confident about offering some comforting and settling before you feel the need to offer him a feed. It is best to offer the dream feed at least 3 hours after the last feed before bed. For example, if he feeds at around 7pm then offer the dream feed around 10pm. This feed is offered during sleep because the plan is to move away from Ayaz waking and calling out for you for a feed.

Offering it while he sleeps will be sure the message about crying out for a feed, and having some settling time before feeding, remains clear. It is worth a try and is very easy to find out if it is working or not. If it works he may sleep for a little longer, and you will feel more confident about settling before feeding at the next waking. It is also easy to tell if it is not working because if he doesn't easily drift back to sleep, then it is not right for him at this time. Don't be afraid to try because you can't harm him by offering this late evening feed.

Settling tips

You will need to take it slowly to allow Ayaz to see the pattern of settling that you're changing to. You know just what is in your head, but Ayaz doesn't, and it is best to avoid triggering his separation struggles. Just keep repeating the following so he can experience how you can comfort him so he can adjust little by little:

- Taking Ayaz away from your breast before he is fast asleep is your starting point. He will squirm and fuss, but lift him up over your shoulder and cuddle him so he is not laying in a breastfeeding position. If he is really struggling, allow him to comfort suck until he settles, then take him away from your breast again while he is drowsy but still awake
- Once Ayaz is more able to understand that the cuddle is almost as good as sucking and he calms in your arms more easily, it is time to cuddle him for a shorter time, each time, and to start placing him in his cot less and less drowsy. This way he will begin to experience being settled in the cot without the sleep association of sucking and being cuddled
- Although when placed in his cot, Ayaz is unlikely to feel that is enough. He is not accustomed to being aware of being in his cot before sleeps, so you will need to offer him some comforting to see if he can be calmed enough to drift to sleep
- Realistically this will take a week or more, so please don't expect amazing progression from a baby who has no idea what this new way of sleeping is
- When you place drowsy Ayaz into his cot, he will most likely cry so you can:
  - Kneel down on the floor beside his cot so you are not encouraging him to move up towards you if you are standing, which is what happens when you stand over the cot
  - Offer voice comforting in the form of shhing and occasionally telling Ayaz you are there.

You know it's a big change, but you are there. This also helps you remember this is a big change for Ayaz, and to remain calm and kind

- Try shhing and patting the mattress in a slow rhythmical pattern, as if you were patting his back to calm when you cuddle him
- Mattress patting is less stimulating but offers calming rhythm, however if Ayaz seems to be more comforted by a back rub or nappy pat, that is completely fine to do. It is about finding what calms Ayaz and sticking to it
- If he is not calming, just try quiet singing a little to see if activation of other areas of his brain can help him calm, when he calms, just return to the patting and shhing
- If Ayaz goes quiet, just slow whatever you are doing, and shh or sing more quietly
- If he looks like he is drifting to sleep, then just keep the comforting going (after several days if he is calming, then just slowly stop what you are doing and watch to see if he remains calm – if not, return to the comforting)
- If he is still crying after about 30 seconds of shhing and patting and the singing is not calming him … just pick him up and rock him until calm, once calm put him back in the cot and go back to the start and kneel or sit on the floor beside the cot, down at the mattress level

- Be mindful that if you keep eye contact with him, he is likely to remain engaged with you. It is preferable that you are there, comforting and trying not to be a stimulating, engaging presence, just kind and calm
- If he cries, that is a good time for eye contact if he is keen, to connect and calm him. Be guided by his response. If he is more distressed, try averting your gaze and again monitor his response. This way you are being guided by his needs
- The aim is not to cause distress but rather offer repeated short settlings with the plan being that your soothing will gently help create some distance from the immediate expectation of being fed to sleep
- Of course if Ayaz is not calming after you have tried this a few times, then try cuddling to sleep, but if that is taking a long time or if you are too tired to do that, then feed him to sleep and just be sure you start the same way each time, so place him back into his cot once asleep
- Avoid long settlings because they only distress everyone and that is not the environment we are trying to achieve. I know this is repeated, but I also know you are very tired!

- If Ayaz is calm and just lying in his cot watching you, try walking out of the room and returning if he is becoming distressed and cries out for you. This will show that you will return to him and then

will not continually trigger his separation anxiety
- When you do return to him, repeat the same settling steps so you are making it clear and predictable for Ayaz

The idea is for you to watch Ayaz to see how he responds, so you become aware of what he can tolerate and what he can't. Let him guide you. Look and listen, think … then respond. Be as consistent as possible and monitor his response. Be sure you offer comforting to reduce any distress. Long periods of settling filled with distress will not teach anyone anything except exhaustion and frustration. With brief settling you will be moving away from feeding immediately when he wakes, but you can still offer cuddling or feeding if Ayaz cannot calm. Take it slowly but keep moving forward so that each understanding is built upon. See if you can repeat these settling methods on going to sleep and at each waking, both day and night. Remember, calm and kind will help the change in a way that minimises distress.

My reflections

During the exhaustion of sleep struggles, parents sometimes cannot see that the struggles are rendering the family almost incapable of thinking. The ideas presented helped the family to kindly and compassionately guide their baby into healthier sleep patterns. Approaches that say the only way to promote longer sleep times are through leaving your distressed baby such as controlled crying, or modifications of controlled crying, are misleading. Being gentle achieves the same results with the additional bonus of the parents feeling comfortable about how they are responding to their baby at sleep time.

Sleep associations that involve the parent being constantly present, can become real stumbling blocks at sleep time. Moving the baby progressively away from these allows the baby to become less reliant on the parent and more able to settle back into sleep when moving from one sleep cycle to the next. Also, it's often easier to feed babies to sleep, and if the family is happy, then there is no problem. The struggles arise when the baby is not able to sleep, return to sleep or link one sleep cycle with the next without feeding, and the feed itself is more of a sleep association than for nutrition. Not every baby who relies on feeding to sleep experiences sleep struggles. Every family situation is different so each family will know when things are not working the way they had hoped. What often happens is that babies who have small frequent overnight feeds, have reduced hunger and don't embrace opportunities to learn about foods, or develop an appetite and interest in solid food intake, which is something to watch for.

Update:

Ten days later:

"We are very happy that Ayaz is sleeping much better. He still likes to cuddle sometimes, but if it is taking a long time I put him in his cot and pat on the mattress. He now sometimes puts his hand on my hand as I pat, and he goes to sleep. He even went to sleep with me just sitting beside him doing nothing today and yesterday. He is much happier and is also eating food better. He still does not like the bottle but he is now drinking my milk from a little cup. He is very good at it when we help him. I also dream feed him every night and he sometimes wakes after that and I hear him moving around but he has gone back to sleep. I think the dream feed is helping him a lot. In this week he has only woken at night twice and I fed him because I think he was cold. He is feeding much better because he seems hungry. He wakes at about 6am and is smiling more. He is a different boy. I hear him in his cot and he does not cry for me straight away when he wakes up. Even if he is hungry he has a play first in his cot then calls me. I still sit with him until he falls to sleep at every sleep, but he can sleep now for 2 hours during the day. He went 6 hours without waking two nights ago. We are very happy with him."

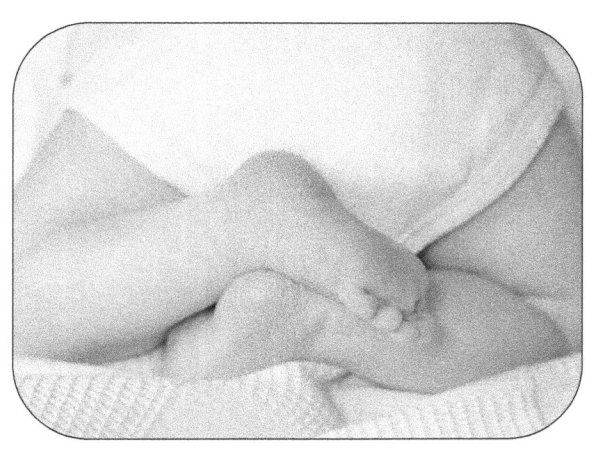

Chapter 7

Charlotte's family story

The story of mother Bec, and baby Charlotte (11 months)

"Charlotte doesn't even sleep soundly when she is in my bed. We are all so sleep deprived now."

"Charlotte has never been a good sleeper. I know I should have been stricter, but I have been a single mother since she was 5 months old. I know I have caused this because I've never forced sleep routines. She seemed to be okay, but since about 6 months her sleep has been getting worse and now it's a mess. I regret not being stricter with getting her into a good routine sooner because I can't get her back into her own cot to sleep now. The only time she will sleep is if I am holding her or lying beside her, so she sleeps in my bed at night. I honestly would be happy with her sleeping with me if she actually slept, but she wakes all the time and she lays on me to get back to sleep. I really don't know how we got to this stage. I am so tired that I get cross with her and I know it's not her fault, it's mine. I have let this happen, and I have tried a few things, but she really hates being in her cot. She just stands there and screams. We also live in a small flat with neighbors who have complained about the noise she makes, so I need to keep her quiet at night. She is generally a happy little girl, but she looks so tired all the time. She goes to day care one day a week and to my parents' house another two days while I work. She doesn't sleep much there either. She will sleep if she is on her grandparents' knees or if they hold her during sleep time in daycare. She sleeps in the pram if my parents take her for a long walk. The hard thing is that she did actually sleep in her cot until she was 6 months old. She's had every sickness going at daycare since she started there. I can't get her to sleep in her cot anymore. I am sure if she were happy in her cot, I would be happy too because I would have more sleep. Sometimes my parents come to my place at night so they can take it in turns sleeping with Charlotte so everyone gets a little bit of sleep. They do this when I am really tired and have to work the next day. I feel awful for letting it get to this stage because I think both Charlotte and I are just always tired now, so I don't have the patience I need and I just end up letting her sleep with me. If she slept quietly I would happily leave her in my bed until she was ready to go to her own bed, but the way it is now, nobody is getting much sleep. She has a bottle at each sleep time, but she doesn't have any more through the night now. I stopped that when she was 9 months old. Not sure if you need to know but her dad left us when she was 5 months old and went overseas. We haven't seen him since. That was a hard time but both my parents and his parents have been wonderful to us, and Charlotte loves all her grandparents, so in that way we are lucky. I don't expect miracles but anything would be better than where we are at now."

There are some key things to think about here:
- Self-regulation
- Transitioning from bed sharing to cot
- Preparation for bed
- Expectations
- Sleep tips

Self-regulation

We hear the term around a lot but what self-regulation refers to in simple terms is the baby's ability to adapt to experiences and control their responses to those experiences [48]. No matter what age, babies and children are always adapting and re-adjusting to the type and volume of incoming information they receive. They are constantly recalibrating to be sure they don't become overwhelmed. Initially, babies are not very sophisticated in their ability to self-regulate, and that is why they need so much assistance from in-tune parents to help.

When parents respond to babies, the babies are building the brain connections that support their understanding of the world, including how to manage intense emotions. Parents offer a form of co-regulation when they help babies experience calming when over-aroused. Repetition of the experience of being regulated allows the brain circuitry to build strong connections that support the growth of self-regulation. Over time the parent can allow a baby and child more and more autonomy in the regulation process, and so this co-regulation process relies less on the parent as the baby develops their own self-regulation capacity. As they grow, they learn to regulate themselves more, but when a baby is 6 months of age their ability to self-regulate without assistance is limited [50,51,52,53,54].

So your decision not to insist Charlotte had to be placed into a strict sleep routine was a good one. When Charlotte commenced childcare there would have, no doubt, been a range of new and exciting experiences for her to adjust to. Self-regulation may also have been compromised because of the ongoing illnesses. For these reasons I would like to challenge your thoughts about you causing her current sleeping by not forcing sleep routines. I suspect if you had tried to impose sleep routines, you would have had a much more unsettled little girl. You and Charlotte sound like life changed pretty dramatically at 5 months and for her to have not been really distressed, I suggest is testament to you for helping her recalibrate in the absence of her other parent. At 6 months when illness and daycare came, it is completely understandable that Charlotte would have additional needs for you to support and comfort her. All this taken into account, I still see no reason for your self-blame. If you had tried to create a strict routine at that time, that would have had the potential to cause significant distress. Again, I congratulate you on your decision. Your baby has had access to you and what sounds like a very caring extended family and it is because of that you have probably protected her from being totally overwhelmed.

So in terms of co-regulation, I feel you have offered Charlotte appropriate care experience in that you have not insisted she be separated from you at times when there have been additional emotional and physical challenges.

Transitioning from bed-sharing to cot

As you rightly say, where your baby sleeps is a personal family choice and your choice to move Charlotte to her bed seems sensible in your situation because she is so unsettled when she sleeps with you, and neither of you are sleeping. Moving Charlotte back into her own cot will be a big shift for you both and I wonder if it would be at all possible that you moved either her cot to your room if it is not already there. Would you consider sleeping in the same room as her for a while as she adapts? This will allow Charlotte some adjustment time, and after she is happily sleeping in her cot, then you can reconsider those sleeping arrangements.

The reason I say this is because Charlotte has had close bodily contact with you and others during her sleep and taking that away suddenly may be too challenging for her physically and emotionally. If you are nearby, you can place her cot near your bed and maybe even place your arm in the cot to soothe her if she is unsettled for a few nights. Also I think that will also help you be less worried about your neighbors' concerns if you are near her. You may find there are times she understands she is okay to be in her cot near you, and there will be other times she becomes distressed. The steps below are to help with that transition.

Preparation for bed

You probably have a great pattern in place so this is more to consolidate that idea. However, if you don't, then it is a good idea to have something that helps Charlotte see that it is getting near sleep time. The wind down time is very important to help her calm in preparation for sleep. You might find that the days she is in care, she is ready for bed earlier because she has used so much energy; physically, socially and emotionally. Often overtired babies rev up and look active and not tired, but they are easily distressed and what they need is bed time rather than distraction that keeps them awake longer.

Another thing we tend to do is delay sleep time a little if it is really hard, so my recommendation is into bed earlier rather than later, if you can. In preparation for bed, book reading is great because it gives the baby physical contact as well as the shared time together. It can be surprising how powerful reading a book together can be for helping you and your baby connect in a meaningful way [55].

The following are some of the signs you might see that give you a clue that Charlotte is getting tired; fussy, grizzling, intolerant of things she normally loves, disinterest in her toys or seemingly getting bored quickly, she might look pale and darkened areas under her eyes might appear. If you don't act on these signs, Charlotte will become increasingly fussy and unhappy and may become really distressed for no particular reason, and may be very difficult to calm. Watch Charlotte closely to see if there is something else you notice. Maybe she rubs her eyes, yawns or just looks really disinterested in her environment. Whatever it is, this is certainly her body saying it is sleep time, and acting on those signs will avoid the struggles that inevitably come with settling overtired babies for sleep.

Something else to consider is that screens have been shown to arouse babies and children, so it is recommended no screens before bedtime. There is not a researched time frame but considering it takes children about half an hour to calm down after using screens, it would make sense to have no TV, or handheld devices for around half before bed time [56]. A darkened room helps give the sleep message, so even if you sit in a room with low lighting during pre-sleep quiet time, that may be helpful.

Rhythm can be soothing and quite mesmerising for babies, so either singing or humming while patting Charlotte, or snuggling her in a swaying, rocking type of slow dance to give her arousal system a chance to calm for sleep time. Anything that induces calm is helpful.

I don't know if you use a sleeping bag, but the 'arms out ones' are really helpful in keeping babies warm even if they have moved on top of their bedding. Also, when a baby finally does go to sleep and you are not in the room, you will be less tempted to take that leap of faith of creeping back into the room to be sure the blankets are covering her. If you have ever tried to sneak into the room of a baby who is learning to sleep, it's a pretty risky business. That is a big plus for a sleeping bag. Also it is good to remember that for Charlotte, sleeping with you has been like sleeping on and beside a heater, because of your body heat she has been snuggling into. So rather than warm her room, the sleeping bag fits the bill perfectly. Remember though, if Charlotte ends up back in your bed through the night, she is either better laying on top of your bedding or remove her sleeping bag if she insists on being under the bed clothing to avoid overheating.

Another critical component of sleep preparation is timing. In fact, timing is everything. Overtired babies do not only struggle to settle, they are very easily over-aroused and crying and hysterics follow in the footsteps of being overtired. Babies and parents have to work much harder to find sleep once a baby is overtired. If you have trouble seeing Charlotte's tired signs then keep an eye out for her looking pale, rubbing her eyes or snuggling her face into you, staring unfocussed for short times or just getting grizzly. The hard thing is if you miss the early signs, then by the time she is yawning and really grumpy, she will be very close to being overtired. Some babies when overtired seem to become more active and she may look like she is not tired at all. So you then let her play a little longer, but it is not normal behavior, you are seeing. Overtired babies are more revved up and what some parents call hyperactive, then suddenly the baby shows what overtired really looks like and is finding it impossible to calm. Inconsolable tears often follow this hyped, overtired phase. Being watchful for those signs can save a lot of sleep time grief.

Expectations

When everyone is tired and people are trying to help, this can lead to confusion and a lack of confidence in parenting. There are some simple things to remember in terms of babies and sleep needs and times. Every child is different in how much sleep they need, just like adults. Some adults function on very few hours of sleep and others need more, much more. It is that crazy situation with babies where all we want is for them to sleep, and often they resist it. It seems such an irony that babies resist sleep and parents crave it. It is so hard to understand why babies don't take every single opportunity to sleep, like an adult would if given the chance. It is good to be mindful that there is no intent on the baby's behalf to interfere with your sleep.

Every few years there is a study published that identifies 'normal sleep patterns' for babies. It is great to have a guide, but what is evident in those works it that there is enormous variation in what is normal, and the hours identified represent the majority of babies, but not all fit into the majority. Rule of thumb is to watch your baby, read the gestures and signs that this brain, this body, right now is preparing for sleep. That is when a baby should sleep; when the body needs it. Studies of 'normal' sleep and waking patterns have shown that it is completely normal for some babies to wake through the night ... until and often beyond 18 months of age if not longer [57]. Of course, we would love to have babies sleeping through the night from 2 weeks of age, so WE can sleep, but that is not how babies work. They are not adults and they need to wake overnight for nutrition and sometimes reassurance.

In your case Bec, you sound very realistic, not expecting Charlotte to sleep through the night, because she may well be one of those babies who naturally progresses to reduce her overnight wakings until she is into her second year of life. We often feel pushed to rush them to sleep though because everyone tells stories of babies who sleep through, as if that's a badge of honor. Some babies actually need to wake and be cared for as they grow and develop. Adults often crave sleep because sleep deprivation can take its toll [58]. However, if a baby wakes infrequently, feeds and returns to sleep readily, that is probably quite a normal waking pattern for them. Overnight waking is a problem when the wakings are long and frequent, and over time, are not reducing. Then that is time for change, for sure.

After making some changes to your responses to Charlotte's waking, she may well still wake for some reassurance. If you offer it, try not to have her rely on you to be with her to return to sleep all the time. She is more likely to just progress through until she no longer wakes. Staying realistic and remembering babies have different sleep requirements and waking patterns to adults can be helpful for some parents to help them remain kind and gentle when their baby wakes overnight. For now, Charlotte will need your company to help her make this transition to her own bed. The most important thing is to read how much she needs you. Look for her signs and monitor how she responds to your comforting efforts.

Sleep tips

- Sleep time starts with a predictable routine in a low stimulation environment, without screens, that includes some hugs and body contact, which can include book time
- Rhythm is a very effective calmer, so you might like to just cuddle Charlotte and pat her back as you rock from foot to foot, even humming or a quiet song she likes can help soothe her and prepare her for sleep
- When calm, place her in her cot
- Most likely she will protest, and stand up
- You immediately move down low until you are at the cot mattress level
- Place your arm in through the rails and start patting the mattress and shhing
- Initially she will have absolutely no idea what you are doing, so keep the time brief
- I am not sure if she has a dummy, but if so offer it when you see, that she is unable to settle after perhaps 30 seconds or so of shhing
- Also this is the time to lay her down; if you do it immediately she will begin to rely on you to lay her down

- Assess to see if she is calming, if not, move to patting her, and see if that helps soothe her at all
- If so, just keep going; until she sleeps the first few times, but the aim is to reduce your patting when she becomes calm and to leave her in her cot when she is calm. To start with though, just pat and shh quietly
- If you stay with Charlotte and she is tossing and turning in her cot, and unable to settle for sleep, then just walk out of the room and listen to her response
- If she remains the same, then allow her some time to see if she can settle in for sleep. If she is still restless after 5 minutes or so you may find going back into her to give her a little pat to help her soothe may be helpful, because if you leave her too long, she may quickly become overtired
- If she cries, she is calling you back in, so just briefly shh a few times from outside her room so she knows you are nearby, if she is not calming, then go in and go to that same position; low down beside the cot so it is clear you are not picking her up – yet
- Again offer the mattress patting and shhing, as above, but if she doesn't calm pick her up and cuddle her until she is calm
- Once calm place her back into her cot and try again. The idea is to keep settlings short and with minimal distress, and if Charlotte does become distressed then you offer her comforting initially in the cot, then in your arms
- If Charlotte is just not able to respond to your comforting efforts each time you pop her back in

- her cot, then just cuddle her to sleep or put her in bed with you
- Once she is asleep, sound asleep, gently move her back into her cot
- That way, the next time she wakes you can offer some of the settling again. By doing this Charlotte will have the opportunity to repeatedly experience your comforting when she is in her cot, to help her understand the change process
- You may find that Charlotte just cannot calm without body contact because of her experience of lying on you or your parents when she sleeps
- This is the time that you can, if possible, place her cot close to your bed so you can leave your arm through the rails of the cot ... and you get to lay in your own bed. Win:win. This is a starting point to you progressively moving away from Charlotte, yet not expecting her to suddenly understand what you want, and accept it willingly. She will need help
- You may find that trying the settling for just 5 or 10 minutes at a time, will allow you both time to adjust to this new approach to settling for sleep
- If Charlotte does seem to be settled and calm, you can leave her room, and if she instantly cries to call you back, it is a fine line between responding to her cry yet allowing her a moment to try to self-regulate
- For that reason, 3 or 4 cry outs are all that is needed for you to know if she is able to do something to calm herself a little. If you listen to those brief cry outs, and by the 4th cry the intensity is not lessening, then offer her about 5 seconds

of shhing from outside her door so she knows you are near
- If she is not calming to your voice shhing, then go into her
- Again, keep low and start back to the steps above; sitting down low beside her cot.

I will repeat this because sometimes tired parents need to hear it a few times. This settling is not about long periods or intense distress. It is about allowing your baby to experience you supporting them and offering them comfort. If they cannot respond to whatever you are offering, then you need to move to the next step, this is called incremental care, with increasing the care you offer until calm is reached. Long, distressed-filled times of trying to 'put' a baby to sleep is completely different to comforting a baby so they can calm and find sleep. So, keep the settling times short and just repeat them at each waking. Avoid long and distressed episodes.

My Reflections

Exhaustion can interfere with a parent's ability to clearly see what is happening for their baby, which can result in the baby feeling like they need to be asking for more to help them feel like their world is manageable. By a parent thinking about the baby's experience and setting up some steps to help the baby feel there is someone there for them, the baby can then put their energy into just being, rather than needing to be in constant contact with the parent to gain that sense of security and safety. Charlotte is not different to any other baby who is finding their tired parents are not able to be as emotionally available as they need them to be.

Babies need their parents to see their emotions, but not be overwhelmed by them. If the parent can do this, then they reflect the information back to the baby in a way that is less overwhelming. For example, when a baby frantically cries, if a parent can see the distress and even feel it, but not become it, they are more likely to be able to calmly reflect back to the baby that these intense emotions are tolerable to the parent. This then helps the baby experience these feelings and experiences as tolerable.

Many sleep struggles seem to really intensify when exhausted parents are no long able to see the subtle, small gestures, cues and behaviours, and the baby then escalates to express their experiences. What often follows is the baby's brain is not supported with the neural connections that are needed for the ongoing development of self-regulation and social skills, resulting in stress all round. When less tired, parents are more able to be sensitive to the signals and, therefore, offer an appropriate response to the baby's experience. This becomes the synchronous infant-parent relationship which forms the basis of a secure and enduring relationship.

Update:

"Only two weeks in and I'm not sure where to start. I feel teary when I say this because I still can't believe it. Charlotte is in her cot in her room. I am in my bed without her. I miss her but don't miss the little bits of sleep I was getting. The first few days and nights Charlotte didn't want anything to do with her cot so I kept doing the first steps then bringing her into bed with me. I was really tired. About the 3rd or 4th night, I can't remember, after she would go to sleep in my bed I got more determined to get her back into her cot. I would do the steps when she woke. On the 5th night she went to sleep in her cot, and I had my arm in there a bit, and she went straight back to sleep. It was amazing. She has got the idea that I will always come to her if she needs me, but that I only stay until she rolls onto her tummy because that's where she sleeps. The last 3 nights she slept for between 5 to 7 hours without calling out at all. She woke more last night but once I didn't even go to her. I just did the shhh and she went back to sleep without me having to get up to her at all. I still feel sort of sad to be honest, maybe because I should have done this earlier, maybe because I am so tired, and maybe because I am relieved that the nightmare seems to be over, hopefully. My parents are also doing the same steps. They come to my place now and she sleeps in her cot for day sleeps as well. They are really happy too. Mum has started cooking again. You asked what really shifted in me and Charlotte, I think it was that I could really see she needed me and I could see I was so tired and I wasn't giving her that connection to me that she needed with me. She loves book time and so do I. I really think she just wanted someone to be kind at sleep time and I was just grumpy and impatient."

Afterword
Be kind to yourself; allow your intuition to grow

Filter advice. Practise trusting in your 'radar' even if you are deliriously tired. Just run information past your 'does that sound right?' filter. Be wary of those who spend vast amounts of time and energy telling you how to do it better, or telling you how you are doing parenting all wrong. Be aware that they may need to be making you feel bad because they have their own issues and by keeping the focus on you, may redirect the focus to you and deflect it from themselves. Just putting it out there. This may not necessarily be the case, but it is always good to question the motives of someone, especially someone who has a need to make you feel like a bad parent. Of the many parents I meet and know, they are good people doing the very best they can as a new parent. Even if you are not a new parent, and have other children, you are a new parent to your new baby, and because each baby is different, it is worth remembering that this individual baby is new to you.

While on the subject; a word on social media. Facebook and blogs have the potential to offer incredible support for parents because parenting may feel very isolating and lonely. To have a group of 'like mind-eds' can be really supportive. Again, be mindful of those who feel the need to put you down or make you feel you are not doing your best. In fact, if you feel that, just un-friend them or block that group because there are some wonderfully supportive and informative groups out there who can make parenting feel better, and that fit with the different personalities and temperaments within your family. Also, not all that is posted is fact. Some like to tell stories for attention, some need to debrief and some are not representative of the majority of experiences, and can therefore lead you to be fearful of things that are most likely not going to happen to you or your baby. Some like to write about what they wished was happening rather than what is happening in their real world.

It is well known that people are more likely to report negative events than positive, so find a social network who are truly supportive and who give you good ideas and share suggestions without needing to be judgmental of you or your style of parenting.

If you are struggling, find someone who is genuine in their support; be it family or friends, your maternal child and family health nurse or another professional who will respect each individual member of your family and guide you through the tough times in a way that, deep down, feels right for you.

Wishing you peaceful sleep times.

Helen

If you are interested, you may find some of the free articles on my website helpful www.helenstevens.com.au.

Connect to Sleep

Daily sleep hours GUIDE

Please see next page for our guide.

Age	Number of feeds per 24 hours	Awake periods total	No of daytime sleeps	Overnight feeds	Total sleep over 24 hours
0–12 weeks	Anywhere between 10 feeds for a newborn to 6-8 feeds by around 12 weeks of age	Awake after feed for 10 mins for some newborns, and up the 1¼ hours occasionally for 3-month-old	6-10 for a newborn down to around 4 to 5 sleeps per day for a 12-week-old	Yes, often	Around 16 to 22 hrs (ish) in 24 hours, but remember huge variation is normal
3–6 months	Around 6-8 feeds at 3 months to around 5-6 feeds by 6 months of age	1 ½ hours at around 3-4 months up to 2 hours wake time around 6 months	At least 2-3 day sleeps plus a short nap for some babies. With increasing sleep times, overnight	Reducing but maybe at least one feed for some babies at 6 months	15 to 18 (ish) hours in 24 hours

| 6–12 months | Around 5-6 feeds at 6 months to 3 or 4 maybe for a 12-month-old (solids before milk from 9 months) | Around 2 hours of awake time for 6-month-old, up to about 3 hours for a 12-month-old | 6-month-old may have 2 long sleeps and maybe a nap, a 12-month-old may have 2 sleeps but may reduce to one longer one | Some babies continue to need a feed, which is completely fine. There is no fixed time to stop overnight feeds | 14 to 15 (ish) hours |

Every baby is completely different so please use this as a guide only, because there is even huge variation in the research. This guide is to help extremely tired parents to look for tired signs and to act on them, in an effort to prevent babies from becoming overtired. This is a GUIDE ONLY.

References

[1] Baradon, T., Biseo, M., Broughton, C., James, J. and Joyce, A., 2016. The practice of psychoanalytic parent-infant psychotherapy: Claiming the baby. Routledge.

[2] Swain, J.E., Lorberbaum, J.P., Kose, S. and Strathearn, L., 2007. Brain basis of early parent–infant interactions: psychology, physiology, and in vivo functional neuroimaging studies. Journal of child psychology and psychiatry, 48(3-4), pp.262-287.

[3] Bowlby, J., 1973. Attachment and loss, vol. II: Separation (Vol. 2). New York: Basic books.

[4] Stern, D.N., 1995. The motherhood constellation. A unified view of parent-infant psychotherapy.

[5] http://developingchild.harvard.edu Centre of the Developing Child. Harvard University

[6] Zeanah, C.H. ed., 2009. Handbook of infant mental health. Guilford Press.

[7] Trevarthen, C., 2001. Intrinsic motives for companionship in understanding: Their origin, development, and significance for infant mental health. Infant Mental health journal, 22(1-2), pp.95-131.

[8] Leerkes, E.M., Blankson, A.N. and O'Brien, M., 2009.

Differential effects of maternal sensitivity to infant distress and nondistress on social-emotional functioning. Child development, 80(3), pp.762-775.

[9] Landry, S.H., Smith, K.E. and Swank, P.R., 2006. Responsive parenting: establishing early foundations for social, communication, and independent problem-solving skills. Developmental psychology, **42(4)**, **p.627**.

[10] Middlemiss, W., Stevens, H., Ridgway, L., McDonald, S. and Koussa, M., 2017. Response-based sleep intervention: Helping infants sleep without making them cry. Early Human Development, 108, pp.49-57.

[11] Middlemiss, W., Granger, D.A., Goldberg, W.A. and Nathans, L., 2012. Asynchrony of mother–infant hypothalamic–pituitary–adrenal axis activity following extinction of infant crying responses induced during the transition to sleep. Early human development, 88(4), pp.227-232.

[12] Winnicott, D.W., 1960. The theory of the parent-infant relationship. The International journal of psycho-analysis, 41, p.585.

[13] Bowlby, J., 1958. The nature of the child's tie to his mother. The International journal of psycho-analysis, 39, p.350.

[14] Haley, D.W. and Stansbury, K., 2003. Infant stress and parent responsiveness: regulation of physiology and behavior during still-face and reunion. Child development, 74(5), pp.1534-1546.

[15] Tronick, E., 2007. The neurobehavioral and social-

emotional development of infants and children. WW Norton & Company.

[16] Grych, J.H., 2002. Marital relationships and parenting. Handbook of parenting, 2, pp.203-225.

[17] Stern, D.N., 1983. The Early Development of Schemas of Self, Other, and 'Self With Other.'. Reflections on self psychology, pp.49-84.

[18] Beebe, B. and Lachmann, F.M., 1988. The contribution of mother-infant mutual influence to the origins of self-and object representations. Psychoanalytic psychology, 5(4), p.305.

[19] Bretherton, I. and Munholland, K.A., 1999. Internal working models in attachment relationships: A construct revisited.

[20] Winnicott, D.W., 1947. Hate in the countertransference (p. 194-203). London: Tavistock.

[21] Bowlby. J., 1988. A Secure Base. Routledge.

[22] http://cosleeping.nd.edu/safe-co-sleeping-guidelines

[23] https://www.breastfeeding.asn.au/bfinfo/breastfeeding-co-sleeping-and-sudden-unexpected-deaths-infancy

[24] Ainsworth, M.S., 1989. Attachments beyond infancy. American psychologist, 44(4), p.709.

[25] Feldman, R., Weller, A., Leckman, J.F., Kuint, J. and Eidelman, A.I., 1999. The nature of the mother's tie to her infant: Maternal bonding under conditions of proximity,

separation, and potential loss. Journal of Child Psychology and Psychiatry, 40(6), pp.929-939.

[26] Lieberman, A.F., Silverman, R. and Pawl, J.H., 2000. Infant-parent psychotherapy: Core concepts and current approaches. Handbook of infant mental health, 2, pp.472-484.

[27] Ainsworth, M.S., 1991. Attachments and other affectional bonds across the life cycle. Attachment across the life cycle, pp.33-51.

[28] Schore, A.N., 2015. Affect regulation and the origin of the self: The neurobiology of emotional development. Routledge

[29] Meins, E., 2013. Security of attachment and the social development of cognition. Psychology press.

[30] Feldman, R., 2007. Parent–infant synchrony and the construction of shared timing; physiological precursors, developmental outcomes, and risk conditions. Journal of Child psychology and Psychiatry, 48(3-4), pp.329-354.

[31] Crockenberg, S. and Leerkes, E., 2000. Infant social and emotional development in family context.

[32] Nugent, K., 2011. Your baby is speaking to you: A visual guide to the amazing behaviors of your newborn and growing baby. Houghton Mifflin Harcourt.

[33] Barnard, K.E., 1976. NCAST II learners resource manual. Seattle, WA: NCAST.

[34] Swain, J.E., Kim, P. and Ho, S.S., 2011.

Neuroendocrinology of parental response to baby-cry. Journal of neuroendocrinology, 23(11), pp.1036-1041

[35] Kelly, K., Slade, A. and Grienenberger, J.F., 2005. Maternal reflective functioning, mother–infant affective communication, and infant attachment: Exploring the link between mental states and observed caregiving behavior in the intergenerational transmission of attachment. Attachment & human development, 7(3), pp.299-311.

[36] Galland, B.C., Taylor, B.J., Elder, D.E. and Herbison, P., 2012. Normal sleep patterns in infants and children: a systematic review of observational studies. Sleep medicine reviews, 16(3), pp.213-222.

[37] Gay, C.L., Lee, K.A. and Lee, S.Y., 2004. Sleep patterns and fatigue in new mothers and fathers. Biological Research for Nursing, 5(4), pp.311-318.

[38] Emotional regulation Calkins, S.D. and Hill, A., 2007. Caregiver influences on emerging emotion regulation. Handbook of emotion regulation, 229248.

[39] http://developingchild.harvard.edu Centre of the Developing Child. Harvard University

[40] Schore, A.N., 2001. Effects of a secure attachment relationship on right brain development, affect regulation, and infant mental health. Infant mental health journal, 22(1-2), pp.7-66.

[41] Tronick, E. and Beeghly, M., 2011. Infants' meaning-making and the development of mental health problems. American Psychologist, 66(2), p.107

[42] Crockenberg, S. and Leerkes, E., 2000. Infant social and emotional development in family context.

[43] Lieberman, A.F., Padrón, E., Van Horn, P. and Harris, W.W., 2005. Angels in the nursery: The intergenerational transmission of benevolent parental influences. Infant mental health journal, 26(6), pp.504-520.

[44] Fraiberg, S., Adelson, E. and Shapiro, V., 1975. Ghosts in the nursery: A psychoanalytic approach to the problems of impaired infant-mother relationships. Journal of the American Academy of Child Psychiatry, 14(3), pp.387-421.

[45] http://cosleeping.nd.edu/safe-co-sleeping-guidelines

[46] http://www.sidsandkidsvic.org/safe-sleeping-education

[47] Carskadon, M.A. and Dement, W.C., 2005. Normal human sleep: an overview. Principles and practice of sleep medicine, 4, pp.13-23

[48] https://helenstevens.com.au/help-for-parents/overtiredness-in-babies-toddlers

[49] Thompson, R.A. and Limber, S.P., 1990. "Social Anxiety" in Infancy. In Handbook of social and evaluation anxiety (pp. 85-137). Springer US.

[50] Papoušek, M. "Disorders of behavioral and emotional regulation: Clinical evidence for a new diagnostic concept." Disorders of behavioral and emotional regulation in the first years of life (2008): 53-84.

[51] Porges, S.W., 2011. The Polyvagal Theory: Neurophysiological Foundations of Emotions, Attachment,

Communication, and Self-regulation (Norton Series on Interpersonal Neurobiology). WW Norton & Company.

[52] Cozolino, L., 2014. The Neuroscience of Human Relationships: Attachment and the Developing Social Brain (Norton Series on Interpersonal Neurobiology). WW Norton & Company.

[53] Siegel, D.J., 2012. Pocket Guide to Interpersonal Neurobiology: An Integrative Handbook of the Mind (Norton Series on Interpersonal Neurobiology). WW Norton & Company.

[54] Bernier, A., Carlson, S.M. and Whipple, N., 2010. From external regulation to self-regulation: Early parenting precursors of young children's executive functioning. Child development, 81(1), pp.326-339

[55] Vally, Z., Murray, L., Tomlinson, M. and Cooper, P.J., 2015. The impact of dialogic book-sharing training on infant language and attention: a randomized controlled trial in a deprived South African community. Journal of Child Psychology and Psychiatry, 56(8), pp.865-873.

[56] Zimmerman, F.J., Christakis, D.A. and Meltzoff, A.N., 2007. Television and DVD/video viewing in children younger than 2 years. Archives of Pediatrics & Adolescent Medicine, 161(5), pp.473-479.

[57] Weinraub, M., Bender, R.H., Friedman, S.L., Susman, E.J., Knoke, B., Bradley, R., Houts, R. and Williams, J., 2012. Patterns of developmental change in infants' nighttime sleep awakenings from 6 through 36 months of age. Developmental psychology, 48(6), p.1511.

[58] Meltzer, L.J. and Mindell, J.A., 2007. Relationship between child sleep disturbances and maternal sleep, mood, and parenting stress: a pilot study. Journal of Family Psychology, 21(1), p .67.

About the Author

Helen is well known in the professional and parenting world for her ability to translate her knowledge to baby and toddler sleep problems. She has worked alongside families struggling with baby and toddler dysregulation for over 20 years. As a registered nurse, midwife and maternal and child nurse qualified in infant mental health, Helen brings research and findings together in a way that makes the information accessible to both parents and professionals. Through webinars, training and conferences for academics to parenting groups, Helen's message to consider the infant experience is well regarded. As researcher and writer her focus on family mental health and wellbeing has resulted in her compassionate and informed approach to infant sleep being recognised worldwide.

www.ingramcontent.com/pod-product-compliance
Lightning Source LLC
Chambersburg PA
CBHW041318110526
44591CB00021B/2835